The Hands-On Guide for House Officers

ANNA DONALD
BA, BM, BCh (Oxon), MPP (Harvard)

MICHAEL STEIN
MB ChB, BSc (Hons) (UCT), D Phil (Oxon)

b

**Blackwell
Science**

© 1996 by
Blackwell Science Ltd
Editorial Offices:
Osney Mead, Oxford OX2 0EL
25 John Street, London WC1N 2BL
23 Ainslie Place, Edinburgh EH3 6AJ
350 Main Street, Malden
  MA 02148 5018, USA
54 University Street, Carlton
  Victoria 3053, Australia
10, rue Casimir Delavigne
  75006 Paris, France

Other Editorial Offices:
Blackwell Wissenschafts-Verlag GmbH
Kurfürstendamm 57
10707 Berlin, Germany

Blackwell Science KK
MG Kodenmacho Building
7–10 Kodenmacho Nihombashi
Chuo-ku, Tokyo 104, Japan

The right of the Author to be identified
as the Author of this Work has been
asserted in accordance with the
Copyright, Designs and Patents Act 1988.

First published 1996
Reprinted with corrections 1998 (twice),
1999 (three times), 2000

Set by Excel Typesetters Co., Hong Kong
Printed and bound in Great Britain
at the Alden Press Limited,
Oxford and Northampton

The Blackwell Science logo is a
trade mark of Blackwell Science Ltd,
registered at the United Kingdom
Trade Marks Registry

DISTRIBUTORS

Marston Book Services Ltd
PO Box 269
Abingdon
Oxon OX14 4YN
(*Orders*: Tel: 01235 465500
      Fax: 01235 465555)

USA
Blackwell Science, Inc.
Commerce Place
350 Main Street
Malden, MA 02148 5018
(*Orders*: Tel: 800 759 6102
          781 388 8250
      Fax: 781 388 8255)

Canada
Login Brothers Book Company
324 Saulteaux Crescent
Winnipeg, Manitoba R3J 3T2
(*Orders*: Tel: 204 837-2987)

Australia
Blackwell Science Pty Ltd
54 University Street
Carlton, Victoria 3053
(*Orders*: Tel: 03 9347 0300
      Fax: 03 9349 5001)

A catalogue record for this title
is available from the British Library

ISBN 0-86542-921-9 (BSL)
ISBN 0-86542-759-3 (IE)

Library of Congress
Cataloging-in-Publication Data

Donald, Anna.
  The hands-on guide for house officers/
Anna Donald, Michael Stein.
    p. cm.
  Includes bibliographical
references and index.
  ISBN 0-86542-921-9
  1. Residents (Medicine)—
Handbooks, manuals, etc.
2. Medicine—Handbooks, manuals,
etc. I. Stein, Michael. II. Title.
RA972.D66   1996
616—dc20   95-50825
                              CIP

For further information on
Blackwell Science, visit our website:
www.blackwell-science.com

Contents

Introduction, xi

How to use this book, xii

Acknowledgements, xiii

Abbreviations, xiv

1 Starting up, 1
Panic?, 1
  people to help you, 1
  three basic tips, 2
Other useful start-up
    information, 2
  books, 2
  dress, 2
  equipment, 3
  geography, 3
  ward rounds, 4
  discharging patients, 5
  work environment, 5

**2 Getting organized (Four
lists and a folder), 7**
Personal folder, 7
Keeping track of patients
    (List 1), 7
List of things to do (List 2), 8
Phone numbers (List 3), 8
Firm timetable (List 4), 8

3 Paperwork, 10
Patient notes, 10
Accident forms, 10
Blood forms and requesting
    bloods, 11
Consent, 12
Death and cremation
    certificates, 12

Discharge summaries, 12
Drug charts, 13
Drug prescriptions, 13
Handovers, 13
Hand backs, 13
Referral letters, 13
Self-discharge, 14
Sick notes, 14

**4 Accident and
emergency, 15**
General, 15
Admitting and allocating
    patients, 15
Keeping track of patients, 16
Medicine, 16
Overdose, 16
  treating the patient, 17
  washouts, 19
  Ipecac, 19
  patients refusing treatment, 19
Surgery, 20

**5 Becoming a better
doctor, 21**
Computers, 21
  hardware, 21
  software, 22
  modems, 23
  databases, 23
A bit about the Internet, 23
Keeping up with the
    literature, 24
Evidence-based medicine, 25
Professionalism, 26
Communication, 26
  consultants and senior
    registrars, 27

GPs, 27
nurses, 28
patients, 29
patients' families, 30
Confidentiality, 31
    exceptions to keeping
        confidentiality, 31
Consent, 31

**6 Cardiac arrests and crash
    calls, 32**

7 Common calls, 35
How to use this section, 35
Considerations for all ward
    calls, 35
Abdominal pain, 36
Anaemia, 37
Arrhythmia, 38
    initial management for all
        arrhythmias, 38
    management of specific
        arrhythmias, 39
Calcium, 41
    hypercalcaemia, 41
    hypocalcaemia, 42
Chest pain, 43
Confusion, 44
Constipation, 46
Diarrhoea, 47
Electrocardiograms, 48
    important ECG abnormalities
        to recognize, 51
Eye complaints, 52
    the acute red eye, 52
    sudden loss of vision, 52
    floaters, 53
Falls, 53
Fever, 54
    the immunocompromised
        patient with fever, 56
Fits, 56
Intravenous fluids, 58
    how to prescribe IV fluids, 58

Upper gastrointestinal
    bleeds, 59
    high risk and hypovolaemic
        patients, 60
    low risk patients, 61
Lower gastrointestinal bleeds, 61
Glucose, 61
Gynaecological calls, 62
    vaginal bleeding, 62
    dysmenorrhoea, 63
Haematuria, 64
Headaches, 64
Hypertension, 66
Hypotension, 67
Insomnia, 68
    management with
        benzodiazepines, 69
Itching, 70
Immunocompromised
    (see Fever)
The moribund patient, 70
Nausea and vomiting, 72
Oliguria/anuria (see Urine, low
    output)
Oxygen therapy, 73
    methods of oxygen
        delivery, 73
    pulse oximetry, 74
Phlebitis, 74
    management, 74
Potassium, 74
    hyperkalaemia, 74
    hypokalaemia, 75
Rashes and skin lesions, 76
    disease categories, 77
Red eye (see Eye complaints)
Shortness of breath, 78
The sick patient, 80
Sodium, 80
    hyponatraemia, 80
Transfusions, 81
    blood, 81
    platelet, 82
    reactions, 82

Urine, low output, 83
Basic emergency routine, 84

8 Death and dying, 85
TERMINAL CARE, 85
Communication, 85
   breaking bad news, 85
   ongoing communication with
      dying patients, 86
Pain control, 88
Symptom control, 88
Prescribing for the dying, 88
Support for the dying and
      for you, 88
DEATH, 89
What to do when a patient
      dies, 89
Telling relatives about the
      patient's death, 90
Post mortems, 90
Death certificates, 90
   writing the death certificate,
      90
Referring to the coroner, 91
Cremation forms and fees, 92
   to check for pacemakers, 92
Further reading, 93

9 Drugs, 94
General, 94
Prescribing drugs, 94
   drug charts, 94
   writing prescriptions, 95
   controlled drugs, 95
   verbals, 96
Giving drugs, 96
   drug infusions, 96
   intravenous drugs, 98
Specific drug topics, 99
   antibiotics, 99
   anticoagulation, 100
   anti-emetics, 101
   digoxin, 101
   night sedation, 101

therapeutic drug levels, 102
steroids, 102
Miscellaneous tips, 102

10 Handle with care, 104
Alcoholism, 104
   alcohol withdrawal, 104
Children, 105
Depression, 106
Elderly patients, 106
Haemophiliacs, 107
   taking blood, 107
   for theatre, 107
HIV/AIDS, 107
   taking blood, 107
   HIV testing, 108
Jehovah's Witnesses/Christian
      Scientists, 109
Pregnant women, 109
Sickle cell anaemia, 109
The steroid patient, 110
   side effects of steroids, 110
   withdrawal of steroid
      therapy, 111

**11 Approach to the medical
   patient, 112**
History and examination, 113
Clinical stalemate, 113
Preparing patients for medical
      procedures, 116
   upper gastrointestinal
      endoscopy, 116
   colonoscopy, 117
   flexible sigmoidoscopy, 117
   liver biopsy, 118
   pacemaker insertion, 118
   renal biopsy, 119
Specialist referrals, 120
   cardiology, 120
   endocrinology, 121
   gastroenterology, 122
   haematology, 122
   neurology, 123

renal medicine, 124
respiratory medicine, 124
rheumatology, 125

12   Pain, 126
Pain control, 126
general, 126
Specific analgesics, 126
inhaled drugs, 126
oral drugs, 126
IM/IV opiates, 129
other, 130
Pain control by severity and
underlying condition, 130

13   Practical procedures, 133
general hints, 133
Arterial blood gases, 133
interpreting arterial blood
gases, 136
respiratory disease and arterial
blood gases interpretation,
138
Ascitic tap (see Peritoneal tap)
Bladder catheterization, 138
men, 138
women, 139
Blood cultures, 140
Blood letting, 140
Cannulation, 142
Central lines, 144
insertion of central lines, 144
problems with temporary and
tunneled central lines, 147
using central lines, 147
measuring the CVP, 149
Chest drains, 149
managing a chest drain, 150
how to remove a drain, 151
Electrocardiogram, 151
reading ECGs, 152
Excercise stress test, 152
relative contraindications, 153
the procedure, 153

Glucose tolerance test, 153
Injections, 154
subcutaneous, 154
intramuscular, 155
Intercostal block, 155
Joint aspiration/injection, 155
aspiration, 155
injecting joints, 157
Local anaesthesia, 157
Lumbar puncture, 158
Mantoux test, 161
Nasogastric tubes, 161
Peritoneal tap, 162
Pleural aspiration, 162
Pulsus paradoxus, 165
Respiratory function tests, 165
spirometry, 165
peak expiratory flow rate, 169
Sutures, 169

14   Radiology, 171
Requesting investigations, 171
Minimizing radiation, 171
Common concerns about
X-rays, 171
Pregnancy, 173
Plain films, 173
chest X-rays before surgery,
173
skull X-rays, 173
abdominal films, 173
Contrast studies, 173
intravenous urography, 173
barium swallow, 174
barium meal, 174
small bowel enema, 174
barium enema, 175
Ultrasound, 175
Computerized tomography, 175
general, 175
CT head, 176
Arteriography, 176
Magnetic resonance imaging, 176
Radioisotope scanning, 176

15   Surgery, 178
Routine clerking, 178
Peri-operative prescribing, 181
Consent, 181
    expected side effects after
        surgery, 182
Anaesthetics, 183
Drawing up theatre lists, 184
Marking patients for surgery,
    184
Post-operative care, 184
Complicated patients, 185
    jaundice, 185
    diabetes, 185
    steroid-dependent
        patients, 187
    thyroid surgery, 187
Day surgery, 188
Oro-facio-maxillary surgery, 188
Surgical protocol clerking
    sheet, 189

16   Self care, 191
Accommodation, 191
Alternative careers, 191
Bleep, 192
British Medical Association
    (BMA), 192
Car and insurance, 192
Clothes, 192
Contacting medical colleagues,
    193
Contract and conditions of
    service, 193
    what you need to know about
        your contract, 193
Doctors' mess, 196
    making money for the mess,
        196
Drug representatives, 197
Insurance (room contents), 197
Jobs, 197
    curriculum vitae, 197
    the interview, 198

consultant career
    prospects, 199
locums, 199
Meals, 200
Medical defence, 200
Money, 200
    income protection, 200
    payslip deductions, 201
    pensions, 201
    tax, 202
    telephone banking, 203
Needlestick injuries, 203
    if the patient is known to be
        HIV-positive, 203
    if the patient is known to be
        hepatitis-positive, 204
Not coping, 204
Part-time work, 205
Representation of junior doctors,
    205
Sleep, 205

**Appendix A Useful tests,
numbers and other
information, 207**
Addresses, 207
    poisons information, 207
Barthel Score, 207
Glasgow Coma Scale, 208
Mental Health Act, 208
Mini-mental test score, 209
Notifiable diseases, 209
Results, 210
    haematology, 210
    biochemistry, 210
Useful biochemical
    formulae, 211
Fitness to drive, 212

**Appendix B Diagrams for
explaining procedures to
patients, 215**
A1 The thorax, 215

A2 Coronary arteries, 216
A3 Upper gastrointestinal
    tract, 217
A4 Large intestine, 218
A5 Digestive organs, 219
A6 Female pelvis, 220

A7 Male pelvis, 221
A8 Urinary system, 222
Tunneled central lines (see Fig.
    13.4)

Index, 223

Introduction

Your House Officer year is guaranteed to be one of the big experiences of your life. Free at last from rote learning and endless exams, your house job is intensely practical. The trouble is that the theoretical training in medical school does not usually prepare you for the physical and emotional rigours of hundreds of tasks being thrust upon you around the clock. Similarly, medical textbooks rarely deal with the practical know-how which makes all the difference between clumsy and elegant doctoring.

This book is based on the collective experience of junior doctors who remember only too well the highs and lows of their house job year. It contains information not readily available in standard texts, that will help you to feel competent and confident despite sleepless nights and low blood sugars. It assumes minimal practical know-how. Subjects are listed in alphabetical order within each chapter. A detailed index is also provided for rapid reference.

Whatever you do, keep your head up and keep smiling. Hospitals are funny places. Lots of people love their house job; we hope you are one of them. Take care and good luck!

A.K.D.
M.L.S.

How to use this book

This book is designed as a user-friendly manual. We would recommend skimming through it when you first buy it, and then referring to relevant sections for particular problems that you come across.

This book provides standard algorithms for diagnosis and management of clinical problems that worked for us and our colleagues, in different settings throughout Britain. Please don't follow our instructions slavishly. We realize that every firm has its own way of doing things and that there may be more appropriate algorithms for specialist wards or unusual situations. Like a recipe book, feel free to scrawl in the margins to make it more usable for you. We have included some blank pages at the back for extra notes. We want to emphasize that this book is not the *Oxford Textbook of Medicine*, so please don't expect to find the 337 causes of tropical swollen legs here!

To keep the book compact and maximally relevant to what you need, we have not attempted to replicate the *BNF*. While we do suggest drugs where relevant, we realized from our own experience that the safest and most efficient way to prescribe drugs is to use the *BNF* in conjuction with your hospital's drug formulary.

Finally, if you discover a better way of doing something, please let us know. A card is included in the book for future suggestions. If we can use your suggestion, you will be acknowledged in the next edition of the book.

Acknowledgements

This book is dedicated to Uncle Ivan Harris and to Bruce, Janet and Tom Donald, for the support and love that made writing this book possible.

There are many people we wish to thank: Ian Crossley for his support and repeated reading of draft manuscripts; Ruariridh Milne for his brilliant ideas, and Solly Benatar, Muir Gray, Tony Hope, Lionel Opie, Antony Rosen, David Sackett and Basil Shepstone for their inspiration in practising medicine. We especially want to thank doctors and nurses at the John Radcliffe Hospital and Glasgow Royal Infirmary for their teaching, and humane and rigorous approach to clinical practice.

We would like to thank Deborah Castle, Matt Collins, Helen Dignum, Andy Eynon, Nicholas Fleming, Judy Mead, Joe Rosenthal, and Wim de Villiers for editing, ideas and contributions from their experience in NHS hospitals and health authorities. We don't know what we would have done without Andy's attention to detail and green ink! Helen Dignum wrote most of the chapter on Self care, read and re-read draft manuscripts and contributed her own hints and corrections to most chapters. Thanks also to Chris Glynn for his contribution to the chapter on Pain control and for his enthusiasm, and to Derek Crook for his generosity and encouragement. Many thanks to Satish Keshav, a true gentleman, scholar and friend, who made invaluable suggestions and wrote the section Clinical Stalemate.

Special thanks to Lisa Stein, for listening without criticizing. To Hyme, Jenny and Nicholas Rabinowitz, for their love and friendship. To Oliver and Rosemary Russell for years of love, care and encouragement, with this book and everything else.

We would also like to thank our dear friends who made suggestions, encouraged, fed and watered us throughout the course of this book: Elleke Boehmer, Wim and Katherine deVilliers, Elizabeth Jardine, Steve Matthews, Sarah Nuttall, Joel, Ai-Zhen and Sara Tatelman.

Finally, to Michael Anderson for his generosity and love, not to mention the chess, tips on grammar and daily care that kept the wheels turning in the last stages of the manuscript.

Fifty per cent of the authors' royalties for this book are donated to the University of Cape Town Medical School.

Abbreviations

We include a long list of abbreviations to aid reading medical notes and for reference throughout this book.

μg	micrograms
−ve	negative
+ve	positive
A&E	Accident and Emergency
ABC	Airway, Breathing, Circulation
ABG	arterial blood gases
ac	ante cibum (before food)
ACE	angiotensin-converting enzyme
ACTH	adrenocorticotrophic hormone
ADH	antidiuretic hormone
AF	atrial fibrillation
AFB	acid-fast bacillus
AIDS	acquired immunodeficiency syndrome
ALP (alk phos)	alkaline phosphatase
ALT	alanine aminotransferase
ANA	antinuclear antigen
ANCA	antineutrophil cytoplasmic antigen
ANF	antinuclear factor
APTT	activated partial thromboplastin time
ARC	AIDS-related complex
ARDS	adult respiratory distress syndrome
ARF	acute renal failure
ASAP	as soon as possible
ASD	atrial septal defect
ASOT	antistreptolysin O titre
AST	aspartate transaminase
ATN	acute tubular necrosis
AV	atrioventricular
AVCs	additional voluntary contributions
AXR	abdominal X-ray (plain)
Ba	barium
BBB	bundle branch block
bd	bis die (twice per day)
bHCG	beta-human chorionic gonadotrophin
BMA	British Medical Association
BMJ	*British Medical Journal*
BNF	*British National Formulary*
BP	blood pressure
bpm	beats/minute
C&E	creatinine and electrolytes
Ca	carcinoma
Ca	calcium
CABG	coronary artery bypass graft
CBD	common bile duct
CCF	congestive cardiac failure
CCU	cardiac care unit
CEA	carcino-embryonic antigen
CFC	complement fixation test
CI	contraindications
CK	creatinine kinase
CK-MB	creatine kinase cardiac isoenzyme
CLL	chronic lymphocytic leukaemia
CML	chronic myeloid leukaemia
CMV	cytomegalovirus
CNS	central nervous system

COAD	chronic obstructive airways disease	FEV_1	forced expiratory volume in first second
CPR	cardiopulmonary resuscitation	FFP	fresh frozen plasma
		FOB	faecal occult blood
CRF	chronic renal failure	FSH	follicle stimulating hormone
CRP	C-reactive protein		
CSF	cerebrospinal fluid	FVC	forced vital capacity
CT	computerized tomography	Fx	family
CV	curriculum vitae	g	gram(s)
CVA	cerebrovascular accident	G&S	group and save
CVP	central venous pressure	G6PD	glucose-6-dehydrogenase
CVS	cardiovascular system	GBM	glomerular basement membrane
CXR	chest X-ray		
D&V	diarrhoea and vomiting	GCS	Glasgow Coma Scale
DDAVT	desmopressin	GFR	glomerular filtration rate
DIC	disseminated intravascular coagulation	GGT	gamma-glutamyl transferase
DIP	distal interphalangeal	GH	growth hormone
DKA	diabetic ketoacidosis	GI (GIT)	gastrointestinal
dl	decilitre(s)	GKI	glucose, potassium and insulin
DM	diabetes mellitus		
DOA	date of admission	GMC	General Medical Council
DOB	date of birth	GN	glomerulonephritis
DOD	date of death	GP	general practitioner
DoH	Department of Health	GT	glutamyl transferase
DVLC	Driver and Vehicle Licensing Centre	GTN	glyceryl trinitrate
		GTT	glucose tolerance test
DVT	deep venous thrombosis	GU	genito-urinary
DXT	radiotherapy	HB	heart block
EBV	Epstein–Barr virus	Hb	haemoglobin
ECG	electrocardiogram	HBsAg	hepatitis B surface antigen
EDTA	ethylene diamine tetra-acetic acid	Hct	haematocrit
		HDL	high density lipoprotein
EEG	electroencephalogram	HDU	high dependency unit
ELISA	enzyme-linked immunosorbent assay	Hep	hepatitis
		HiB	*Haemophilus influenzae* B vaccine
EM	electron microscope		
ENT	ear, nose and throat	HIV	human immunodeficiency virus
ERCP	endoscopic retrograde cholangiopancreatography		
		HLA	human leukocyte antigen
ESR	erythrocyte sedimentation rate	HOCM	hypertrophic obstructive cardiomyopathy
FBC	full blood count	HPC	history of presenting complaint
FDP	fibrin degradation product		

HS	heart sounds	LH	luteinizing hormone
HT	hypertension	LIF	left iliac fossa
IBD	inflammatory bowel disease	LMN	lower motor neurone
		LMP	last menstrual period
IBS	irritable bowel syndrome	LOC	loss of consciousness
ICP	intracranial pressure	LP	lumbar puncture
ID	identification	LUQ	left upper quadrant
IDDM	insulin-dependent diabetes mellitus	LV	left ventricle
		LVF	left ventricular failure
Ig	immunoglobulin	LVH	left ventricular hypertrophy
IHD	ischaemic heart disease		
IM	intramuscular	mane	in the morning
INR	international normalized ratio (prothrombin ratio)	MC&S	microscopy, culture and sensitivity
		MCV	mean cell volume
IPPD	intermittent positive pressure ventilation	MDU	Medical Defence Union
		Mg	magnesium
ISDN	isosorbide di-nitrate	mg	milligrams
ITP	idiopathic thrombocytopenic purpura	MI	myocardial infarction
		ml	millilitres
		mmHg	millimetres of mercury
ITU	intensive therapy unit	MND	motorneurone disease
iu (IU)	international unit	MPS	Medical Protection Society
IUCD	intrauterine contraceptive device		
		MRI	magnetic resonance imaging
IV	intravenous		
IVC	inferior vena cava	MRSA	methicillin resistant *Staphylococcus aureus*
IVI	intravenous infusion		
IVU	intravenous urography	MS	multiple sclerosis
JAMA	*Journal of the American Medical Association*	MSK	musculoskeletal
		MST	morphine sulphate tablets
JVP	jugular venous pressure		
K+	potassium	MSU	midstream urine
KCCT	kaolin-cephalin clotting time	N&V	nausea and vomiting
		Na	sodium
KCl	potassium chloride	NB	*nota bene* (note well)
kg	kilograms	NBM	nil by mouth
kPa	kilopascals	*NEJM*	*New England Journal of Medicine*
L	left		
l	litres	NGT	nasogastric tube
LBBB	left bundle branch block	NIDDM	non-insulin dependent diabetes mellitus
LDH	lactate dehydrogenase		
LDL	low density lipoprotein	nocte	in the evening
LFT	liver function test	NR	normal range

NSAIDs	non-steroidal anti-inflammatory drugs	PTH	parathyroid hormone
		PTT	prothrombin time
O&G	obstetrics and gynaecology	PU	peptic ulcer(ation)
		PV	per vaginum
obs	observations	qds	quarte in die somemdum (to be taken four times a day)
OD	overdose		
od	once a day		
PaCO_2	partial pressure of CO_2 in arterial blood	qid	quarte in die (four times a day)
PAN	polyarteritis nodosa	R	right
Pap	Papanicolaou	RA	rheumatoid arthritis
PaO_2	partial pressure of O_2 in arterial blood	RBBB	right bundle branch block
		RBC	red blood cell
PAYE	pay as you earn	RCC	red cell count
PBC	primary biliary cirrhosis	RF	rheumatic fever
pc	post cibem (after food)	Rh	rhesus
PCA	patient controlled analgesia	RTA	renal tubular acidosis/ road traffic accident
PCP	*Pneumocystis carinni pneumonia*	RIF	right iliac fossa
		RS	respiratory system
PCR	polymerase chain reaction	RUQ	right upper quadrant
PCV	packed cell volume	RV	right ventricle
PE	pulmonary embolism	RVF	right ventricular failure
PEFR	peak expiratory flow rate	RVH	right ventricular hypertrophy
PID	pelvic inflammatory disease		
		Rx	treat with
PIP	proximal interphalangeal	SAH	subarachnoid haemorrhage
PM	post mortem		
PMH	past medical history	SBE	subacute bacterial endocarditis
PMT	premenstrual tension		
PN	percussion note	SC (sub cut)	subcutaneous
PND	paroxysmal nocturnal dyspnoea		
		SD	standard deviation
PO	per orum (by mouth)	SE	side effects
PPD	purified protein derivative	SHO	Senior House Officer
PPF	purified plasma fraction	SIADH	syndrome of inappropriate ADH secretion
PR	per rectum		
PRN	pro re nata (as required)	SL	sublingual
pro tem	as required, on an ongoing basis	SLE	systemic lupus erythematosus
		SOA	swelling of ankles
PRV	polycythaemia rubra vera	SOB	shortness of breath
PSA	prostate specific antigen	SR	slow release
PTC	percutaneous transhepatic cholangiography	SR	senior registrar

SRN	state registered nurse	TTA	to take away
stat	statim (immediately)	TTO	to take out
STD	sexually transmitted disease	TU	tuberculin units
		TURP	transurethral retrograde prostatectomy
SVC	superior vena cava		
SVT	supraventricular tachycardia	TURT	transurethral retrograde tumourectomy
SXR	skull X-ray	u (U)	units
T	temperature	U&E	urea and electrolytes
$T_{1/2}$	biological half life	UC	ulcerative colitis
T_3	triiodothyronine	UMN	upper motorneurone
T_4	thyroxine (tetraiodothyronine)	URT	upper respiratory tract
		US	ultrasound
TB	tuberculosis	UTI	urinary tract infection
tds	ter die somemdum (to be taken three times a day)	VF	ventricular fibrillation
		VQ scan	ventilation perfusion scan
TENS	transcutaneous electrical nerve stimulation	VDRL	venereal diseases research laboratory
TG	triglyceride		
TIA	transient ischaemic attack	VLDL	very low density lipoprotein
TIBC	total iron binding capacity		
tid	ter in die (three times a day)	VMA (also HMMA)	vanillyl-mandelic acid
TLC	tender loving care	VSD	ventriculo-septal defect
tPA	tissue plasminogen activator	VT	ventricular tachycardia
		WBC	white blood cell
TPN	total parenteral nutrition	WCC	white cell count
TPR	temperature, pulse and respiratory rate	WPW	Wolff–Parkinson–White syndrome
TRH	thyrotrophin releasing hormone	ZN	Ziehl–Nielsen stain
		Zn	zinc
TSH	thyroid stimulating hormone		

Chapter 1: Starting up

Day one of your house job is rarely the nightmare you think it will be. Half of it is taken up by firm meetings and introductions to the hospital. During the other half you will be introduced to the wards. It's all over before you know what's happening. You are finally a real doctor. And then it's day two and you have to get on with the job. . . .

Panic?

Never panic. The thing that strikes terror into the hearts of day-one House Officers is the thought that they, alone, are expected to battle with disease and death when they have never given an IV drug in their life and don't know how to plug in the paddles of the cardiac arrest trolley. That's if they know where to find it. The ward and hospital are often unfamiliar. The whole thing is enough to give you a nasty rash, which many House Officers do get.

The one thing to remember is: YOU ARE NOT ALONE. You are a modest, essential cog in a vast machine which churns away quite happily whether you know exactly what you're doing or not. You soon will. Nobody expects you to know much on the first day – or even in the first month. And everyone will show you what to do.

People to help you

You are surrounded by people who can help you. They include:

1 Nurses who usually know more about what you are doing than you do, as they have watched and done it for years.

2 Patients who don't mind what you do as long as you are reasonably nice to them, and ensure that they get treated properly and with as little pain as possible.

3 Other doctors who love to demonstrate their skill at just about everything; they are always open to requests for help.

• Problems arise when House Officers do NOT ask for help. If you feel panic rising in your throat, **just ask for help**. This is counter-intuitive for self-reliant medics, but it saves lives (yours and the patient's).

• Attend orientation day for House Officers if the hospital has one. It is useful for finding out what the hospital can do for you.

• If possible contact your predecessors before their last day on the job. They can give you invaluable information about what to expect from your house job (the idea for this book came from a request for help from a new House Officer). In particular, ask them about what your new consultants do and do not like.

• Most people find that they are incredibly tired during their first week of work. Such fatigue usually passes as they get used to the hospital and new routines.

Three basic tips

1 Always take initiative in hospitals. If things aren't working, do something about it. Big institutions can become stupid places to work just because no-one bothers to address things that are clearly going wrong. Figure out a solution and contact whoever is in charge of the problem, whether it be a doctor, nurse, manager or the porter.
2 Similarly, take initiative in managing patients. Present seniors with a plan for your patients rather than just asking them what to do. Thinking strategically makes patient management much more fun.
3 Order your work. When tasks are being fired at you from all directions, priority-setting is really important. Try to learn early on which things are super-urgent and which can wait for more peaceful moments. Despite the hype, there *is* quite a lot of down time in your House Officer year.

Other useful start-up information

Books

Most House Officers read little other than fiction during their house-job. You probably don't need to buy anything you don't already have. A few recommended texts are:

Acute Medicine: Sprigings D. and Chambers J. (1990) Blackwell Science, Oxford. A comprehensive guide to emergencies.
Clinical Examination: Talley N. and O'Connor S. (1996) Blackwell Science, Oxford. This book is great for revising detailed clinical examination.
Oxford Handbook of Clinical Medicine: Hope R.A., Longmore J.M., Hodgets T.J. & Ramrakha P.S. (1993) (new edition due out 1998) Oxford University Press, Oxford. A great pocket reference text for medical and surgical conditions.
Surgical Diagnosis and Management: Dunn and Rawlinson (1991; new edition due out 1998). Blackwell Science, Oxford. A great book for HO and SHO level surgical trainees.
The ECG Made Easy (and its sequel, *The ECG in Practice*): Hampton J. (1997) Churchill Livingstone, Edinburgh. An approachable guide to the mysteries of the ECG.
Junior Doctors' Handbook: Published annually by the BMA, free to members. An excellent summary of your rights and useful information for your early years as a doctor.
Recommended texts for the medical specialties (SHO level texts) include:
Gastroenterology Pocket Consultant: Travis S. (1998) Blackwell Science, Oxford. This book clearly explains gastroenterological problems and procedures which are invaluable for both medicine and surgery, as well as for Membership exams.
Cardiology Pocket Consultant: Swanton (1998) Blackwell Science, Oxford. As for Gastroenterology above.
Lecture Notes on Respiratory Medicine: Brewis (1993) (New edition due out 1998) Blackwell Science, Oxford. Beautiful explanations of the pathophysiology and principles of management of respiratory disease. A very good primer for the Chest Unit job.

Essential Neurology: Wilkinson (1992) Blackwell Science, Oxford. A concise and clearly illustrated guide to clinical neurology. For a more comprehensive guide to differential diagnosis consider *Patten's Neurological Differential Diagnosis* (Springer-Verlag) – a classic text.

Essential Haematology: Hoffbrand and Petit (updated every reprint, the last in 1997) Blackwell Science, Oxford. A superb book!

Essential Endocrinology: Brook and Marshall (1994) Blackwell Science, Oxford. Another very useful primer for an Endocrine Unit job.

There are no particularly good small books for rheumatology or nephrology. We recommend using the appropriate chapter in any medical textbook such as *Medicine*: Axford (1996) Blackwell Science or *Clinical Medicine*: Kumar and Clark (1996) Baillière Tindall, London.

Dress

It is worth bearing in mind that patients often dress up to the nines to 'visit the doctor'. I once watched an elderly woman with deteriorating eyesight, donning high-heeled shoes and lopsided make-up, hobble over the hospital lawn to visit the diabetes clinic. Having always dressed casually, I dressed my best from then on.

• Changing from student to doctor mode can put grave dents into your early pay cheques. If nothing else, buy good quality shoes which will look good and stay comfortable on your 36th hour.

• You may get stained with all sorts of unmentionable substances as an House Officer. *Stain Devils* (from supermarkets and household stores) can remove most things. Soaking garments in cold water and lots of soap, followed by a normal machine wash removes blood stains.

• Most hospitals will reimburse you for dry cleaning bills associated with work-related accidents (such as major blood stains on suits). Phone hospital personnel through the switchboard.

Equipment

Always carry:
1 Pen.
2 Notebook/filofax/piece of paper.
3 Stethoscope.
4 Tourniquet.
5 Torch.
6 Bleep.
7 Loose change for food/drink/newspaper.
8 Ophthalmoscope (if not readily accessible on wards).

For ward rounds and working in casualty, as above plus:
1 White coat.
2 Tendon hammer (preferably collapsible).
3 Wooden spatula.
4 Orange sticks.

• Consider carrying everything in a traveller's pouch.

• Ensure that all equipment is labelled with your name. Hospital wrist bands are good for labelling stethoscopes. Equipment can be engraved.

• House Officers definitely need access to ophthalmoscopes. Ward ophthalmoscopes have an amazing tendency to walk and to run out of batteries. Therefore, it is advisable to acquire your own portable ophthalmoscope, and to look in people's eyes at every opportunity. Welch Allyn markets a veterinary ophthalmoscope ('Pocket Ophthalmoscope 19090') which is portable, relatively cheap and reliable, and little known to medics, as it is advertised for vets, not doctors.

• Ask your ward pharmacist for a couple of aliquots of tropicamide to carry in your top pocket. One to two drops greatly facilitates ophthalmic examination. It takes a few minutes to work. Record the procedure in the notes and tell the nurse. Having failed to do the latter, I was once fast bleeped by a frantic student who thought the patient was coning. Never use tropicamide in patients with history of glaucoma or eye surgery.

Geography

• Get a map of the hospital from reception to help you learn where everything is.
• Specifically, find out the location of: blood gas machines, canteen, casualty, doctors' mess, drink machines, endoscopy, labs for crucial bloods, nuclear medicine, take rooms, wards, X-rays.

Ward rounds

Think of yourself as the ward round producer (much of it *is* theatre). Give yourself 15 minutes preparation time to have everything ready. For each patient be prepared to supply:
1 Patient ID (name, age, DOA, occupation, presenting complaint).
2 Changes in condition and management since last round (with dates of change).

3 Results (any investigations done recently).
4 Assessment (physical, social, psychological).
5 Plan for in-patient management (future investigations, ops, drugs).
6 Plan for discharge (see p. 5).
7 X-rays (ask your seniors which ones to have available).
• Unless the patient asks for relatives to remain present, it is generally a good idea to ask them to leave the room while the team examines the patient (curtains are not sound proof). People will often give you more information if their relatives are not present.
• Ask your registrar which X-rays to have available. Get these from the X-ray department well ahead of time (occasionally the ward clerk arranges this for you).
• Each consultant has up to five pet details that he or she wants to know about each patient. Find out what these are from your predecessor and supply them tirelessly at ward rounds (these could range from occupation to ESR to whether or not the patient has ever travelled to the tropics).
• Never say you've done something that you haven't or argue with colleagues in front of patients.

Social rounds

You need to let the social team know how your patient is going to cope (or not) on discharge.
1 Ask yourself: how is this patient going to manage physically, socially and mentally? Specifically, draw up a list of 'disabilities'. These are things that the patient *cannot do*, for whatever

reason. From the Barthel Activities Index (p. 207), consider bathing, bladder, bowels, dressing, feeding, grooming, mobility, stairs, toilet, transfer.

2 Have relevant patient details ready (see below). Most are available from the medical notes and the front-page admissions sheet. Otherwise try the nurses, nursing notes, the patient, relatives and the GP.

3 If you are required to give a history, try to include the following points:
- Patient ID.
- Prognosis: short and long term.
- GP and admitting rights to local hospitals (usually in the admission sheet at the front of the notes).
- Type of residence and limitations (e.g. stairs).
- Home support and previous reliance on social services.
- Financial status.
- Special problems which need to be addressed (physical, social, mental, legal).
- Questions you want to ask members of the multidisciplinary team to help you plan for discharge of the patient.

4 Go to the meeting with specific questions you want answered. Make sure you come away with 'action points' – not just vague gestures from various team members about your patient's care (this goes for all ward rounds).

5 Translate medical jargon into normal English for social rounds, as some members of the social team may not be fully fluent in medical acronyms.

Night rounds

Always do a night round. This can mean the difference between a relative happy house job and a sleepless nightmare. If you do nothing else, make sure you have checked off the following before going to bed:

1 Analgesia.

2 Fluids.

3 Infusions (make them up and leave them in the fridge; tell the nurses where they are).

4 Sedation.

5 Sign for drugs you have verballed during the evening (p. 96).

6 Ask each team nurse on the night shift if he or she has problems that need sorting out before the morning.

- Start your night round *after* the night nurses' drug rounds have been completed. This is when they identify problems that you need to deal with before going to bed.
- Tell night staff to bleep you if they are concerned about a patient. Paradoxically, this combined with reassurance and information about worrisome patients, cuts down bleeps.
- Inform every team nurse of what to do if a sick patient's condition changes. Sometimes you can set limits for relevant signs (e.g. pulse, CVP, T, BP) beyond which you want to be called. Write these in the notes.
- If bleeped for an apparently trivial matter, try your best not to sound irritated. Be ready to go to the ward, even if only to provide reassurance. Again, paradoxically, this reduces bleeps. If nurses are confident that you will turn up if requested, they will not bleep you ahead of time.
- If your room is a long way from the wards, you can sleep in a side room on the ward. Ask the sister or charge nurse, who will usually oblige, especially if you

offer to strip the sheets in the morning. Point out that you are more readily available if you are sleeping on the ward. You might get brought cups of tea and breakfast in bed!

Discharging patients

Clearing hospital beds is an invaluable skill which will earn you lots of brownie points from virtually everyone. To clear beds effectively:

1 Make plans for people's discharge on the day they arrive. Ask yourself:
  • When will they be likely to leave?
  • What will get in the way of this person going home or being transferred?
  • What can be followed up in clinic?
2 If possible, write discharge summaries (see p. 12) the day *before* the patient leaves to avoid delays.

Work environment

Evidence suggests that upgrading your environment upgrades your work – and you. Old, decrepit NHS hospitals can be very depressing. There are ways you can make your particular corner of it a great place to work, even if the rest of the hospital has miles of yellow peeling paint, dripping pipes and corridors of empty wards.

• There is no crime in asking hospital supplies for better furniture/accesso-ries, like shelving, desk, chairs or bulletin boards. They can always say no.

• Take a plant to work.

• If you have a tiny desk (or no desk), order a better one. Ring hospital supplies and ask if there's a spare one somewhere. Or request a new one. There's nothing like drawers that slide open easily for making paperwork easy. As a doctor with tons of notes to write, you are entitled to a desk of some kind.

• Consider buying a cheap tape deck for your desk +/− earphones. Label it clearly with 'dr.X' – ours have never been stolen. It can do wonders for long winter weekends and nights on call.

• Put postcards/pictures/photos up in your work area. If you don't have a bulletin board, order one from hospital supplies.

• Buy/borrow/beg a spare typewriter if you like writing. In one of my house jobs I had my typewriter permanently on my desk. It made form-filling a lot easier, and enabled me to write letters and stories when I was bored out of my brain on weekend cover.

• Bring decent coffee or cocoa supplies to work. A single-cup cafetiere, some packs of coffee at the back of the ward fridge and jar of your favourite spread can upgrade your existence no end.

• If your ward has photos of the 'ward team' on it, ring Medical Illustration and get them to take photos of the doctors on the ward and put them up too.

Chapter 2: Getting organized (Four lists and a folder)

Keeping track of patients and their details can be the bane of your life as an House Officer. Filling in forms after work is a waste of precious evenings. Fortunately, you can greatly reduce the time you spend chasing paper, patients and results by having four lists and a folder.

Personal folder

A ring binder folder can save days of time on ward rounds and on night call. Unlike a filofax, a folder provides a writing surface at the bedside and an immediate supply of forms during ward rounds, so that you can do all the paperwork during rounds and don't have to come back to the ward later. As well as saving time, using a folder means you are less likely to forget things, because you can do most tasks as soon as they are requested.

How to make a personal folder:
1 You need one A4 ring binder folder with a large plastic pocket inside the front cover, and at least two sets of brightly coloured dividers (WH Smith sells them cheaply).
2 Fill the folder with all the different forms you use during the day, stacking each type of form behind different dividers. Label the dividers. Stuff small forms (e.g. blood forms) in the inside pocket. Useful forms include:
  • Accident forms, blood cards (bio-chemistry, haematology, bacteriology), consent forms, CT cards, discharge forms, drug charts, ECG forms, firm timetable, fluid charts, history sheets, nuclear medicine cards, X-ray forms.
3 If forms are not already hole-punched, you can almost always find a hole-puncher at the ward clerk's desk.
4 Consider sticking a page of phone numbers and/or drug regimes (see p. 8) to the front of your folder for easy reference.

Keeping track of patients (List 1)

This is a hassle. People have devised many complex strategies for ensuring that they have up-to-date details for each patient. However you do it, you need information to hand so that you can answer questions on ward rounds, discuss patients over the phone with GPs, nurses and colleagues, write in the notes and do the discharge summary, and request and find results of investigations. The minimum information for this includes:
• Patient name and hospital number.
• Reason for admission and major details from PMH.
• Main problems now.
• Mainstay of management (e.g. drugs, surgery).
• Recent results.

One way of keeping track of such information is to stick patient labels onto history sheets, leaving a space between each to fill in patient details. Put a line through patients who have been discharged. The labels contain patient ID. A sheet like this can be made up as patients are admitted in casualty, and stored at the front of a personal folder.

List of things to do (List 2)

The simplest ways to keep track of many tasks are to:

1 Keep a daily list on the back of a card that you can update regularly.

2 Keep a small diary to note down requests for days and weeks ahead.

• Write down all requests as soon as you receive them.

• Try subdividing tasks in terms of *where* they have to be done. This enables you to choreograph your movements around the hospital rather than endlessly dashing from one ward to another. For example:

X-ray	give in forms from ward round
	ask Dr A about Mr B's CT
	request barium enema for Mr C

Ward 6A	IV line for Mrs D
	consent Mr E for colonoscopy
Ward 7B	vitamin K for Ms F
	sign verbal for paracetamol

Phone numbers (List 3)

Phone numbers are essential. Making a list early saves a lot of time. You can reduce the list with a photocopier and stick it on the front of your filofax or ward folder for easy reference. From experience, it is easier to find names if the list is strictly alphabetical. Copy or modify Fig. 2.1 if you like.

Firm timetable (List 4)

Hospitals have their own days for doing speciality procedures (such as isotope scans). Colleagues and relevant departments will know what these are.

Get a copy of your team's timetable. Find out from your colleagues what you need to bring for team activities such as X-ray conferences and academic meetings.

Name	Extension	Name	Extension
Anaesthetist		Microbiology	
Bereavement officer		Microbiology on-call	
Biochem		MRI	
Biochem on-call		Nurses' room	
Blood transfusion		OT	
Casualty		Outpatients	
Clotting lab		Pain clinic	
Consultant secretary		Pathology	
CT		Personnel	
Cytopathology		Pharmacist	
Day hospital		Pharmacy-dispensary	
Dermatology referral		Physiotherapy	
Diabetic clinic		Porters	
Doctors' mess		Post mortems	
Doctors' residence		Pulmonary function	
Doctors' room		Records	
Drug information		Registrar	
ECG		Security	
Echo		SHO	
Endoscopy		Social workers	
Gastro referral		SR	
Gerontology referral		Stoma nurse	
Haematology		Take-away	
Haematology on-call		Theatre-reception	
Immunology		Theatre-recovery	
Infection control		Ultrasound	
Library		Wards	
Linen		X-ray	
Lipid lab		X-ray (portable)	
Medical records			

Fig. 2.1 Essential telephone numbers.

Chapter 3: Paperwork

Paperwork is not difficult – just boring. As doctors communicate with many people through forms and notes, it is important that they contain clear information. The most important part of paperwork is writing clear, legible patient notes.

Patient notes

Doctors are legally obliged to write in patients' notes at least once every third day. However it is good practice to write something every day.

1 Always sign notes and print your surname clearly with your bleep number.

2 It is useful to ask two things when writing patient notes:
- Do the notes give enough information to treat the patient when I'm not available?
- Will I be legally covered if these notes were ever before a court?

3 For daily notes, try this checklist (CRAP):

C hange in the patient's condition or management.

R esults of investigations (blood, X-ray and otherwise).

A ssessment of patient's physical and psychological states.

P lan for future (management and discharge).

(SOAP (Subjective, Objective, Assessment, Plan) is another popular acronym. Choose whichever you prefer.)

4 If you're not sure about how to document a patient's condition, flick back through previous notes and see how others approached it – or ask a colleague.

5 It is helpful for subsequent readers if you include the time, date and place (e.g. casualty) in the margin of notes.

6 If you are called to see a patient, briefly document (even if the call was trivial):
- That you saw the patient.
- The time and date.

7 It is foolhardy to write anything in the notes that you would not want the patient or their relatives to read; they have legal access to them.

8 It is perfectly admissable to write 'no change' or words to that effect if nothing much has happened to the patient.

9 Writing how the patient seems to you (e.g. cheerful, sad, fed up) gives a good baseline for future management.

Accident forms

When called to see a patient who has had an accident (e.g. fell out of bed):

1 See the patient as soon as possible. Nurses are legally liable unless they make sure you see the patient.

2 Ask the patient what happened and which part hurts the most. Check:
- T, BP, pulse and respiratory rate.
- Consciousness level (see Glasgow Coma Scale, p. 208).
- Skin for bruising, bleeding, cuts and fractures.
- Bone tenderness and shape for fractures. Frail patients can sustain fractures with remarkably little fuss.

Especially look for hip, wrist and scaphoid fractures. Examine the skull carefully if the patient hits their head. Consult with your senior if there is sign of serious injury or drowsiness — they may request a CT or skull X-ray (see p. 173).

3 Sign an accident form (the nurses will give you one). Filling it in is self-explanatory.

4 Also write in patient's notes. Include:
• Time and date.
• Brief history of accident.
• Brief examination findings.
• That you signed an accident form.

5 If appropriate, ask the nurses to continue to do observations at regular intervals and to contact you if the patient's condition deteriorates.

6 Think about how the accident occurred. If possible, make a plan with the nurses to prevent future accidents.

7 Consider carrying a couple of accident forms in a personal folder (see p. 7); it saves time in the middle of the night.

Blood forms and requesting bloods

• Ask haematologists and biochemists which details on blood cards are essential. Often the cards have spaces for information that is unnecessary.

• Write your bleep and ward number clearly on blood cards so the labs can contact you if necessary.

• Two good times to fill in forms are during the daily ward round and when

Table 3.1 Conditions for which it may be possible to fill out serial forms.

MI on admission	Lipids (only worth doing within 12 hours of infarct; values will change post-MI for 3 months)
Days 1–3	Serial cardiac enzymes
	Serial ECGs
Warfarin initiation	Check the INR at least:
	Every day for 1 week
	Every week for 3 weeks
	Every month for 3 months
	Every 8 weeks after that
Renal failure: daily	Urea
	C&E
TNP: daily	C&E
Mon, Wed, Fri	LFTs, Ca, phosphate, alk phos
Weekly	Mg, Zn, FBC
IV fluids: daily	C&E
Post-op bloods: next day	C&E
	FBC

writing in patients' notes. Having a stack of forms ready saves time.

• Where possible, anticipate patients' blood needs and write forms in bulk. For example, if someone has had a suspected MI, you can write out a stack of cardiac enzyme forms on admission, or on the ward round the next day, for 3 days. Conditions for which it is sometimes possible to fill in serial forms include those shown in Table 3.1.

• Try having a separate plastic bag or a hook or paper clamp for each day of the week in the doctors' office. You can write serial forms at the start of the week and see at a glance who needs what. Alternatively you can stack forms in chronological order on a clip-board.

• One way of keeping track of patients' tests is to write 'FBC' (or whatever) and date under the patient's label in your list of patient details (p. 7).

• If you don't have a phlebotomist, don't despair. Taking bloods in the morning enables you to sort out patients' problems before the ward round and enables you to say good morning to patients on a one-on-one basis. This has remarkable effects on one's efficacy.

Consent (see p. 181)

Death and cremation certificates (see pp. 90, 92)

Discharge summaries (TTO/TTA) (also see Discharging patients, p. 5)

The discharge summary or 'TTO' or 'TTA' (To Take Out or Away) is a sheet that House Officers write for patients to take to their GPs. It enables GPs to con-tinue with outpatient care until the more detailed discharge letter arrives. The letter is usually written by the SHO or registrar but may fall to you. The TTO is also the prescription form that the nurses use to order drugs for the patient to take home with them (although some hospitals provide a separate form for this function).

1 Get the GP's name and address from the patient or the front page of the notes.

2 Complete the TTO before the patient leaves! Include:
  • Patient details.
  • Name of consultant.
  • Name of ward.
  • Diagnosis.
  • Important findings, positive and negative.
  • Treatment given.
  • Treatment on discharge.
  • Follow-up arrangements.
  • What the patient has been told.
  • Your name and bleep number.

3 Patients are often delayed in hospital because TTOs have not been written. Write them as soon as possible so that drugs can be fetched from pharmacy. Patients and nurses will love you for this.

4 Carry a bunch of TTOs on ward rounds so that you can write the TTO on the spot when the decision is made to send someone home. This means that you can check any discharge details with the team, and the form can be sent to pharmacy pronto.

5 Phone the GP on discharge if the patient:
  • Self-discharges.
  • Is in an unstable condition.
  • Has poor home circumstances.
  • Dies.
  • Needs an early visit.

6 Consider phoning the GP if you are discharging a patient with particularly complex or sensitive care needs, such as elderly people living alone or terminally ill patients.

Drug charts (see p. 94)

Drug prescriptions (see p. 94)

Handovers

Before you go home, to bed or away for the weekend you will need to 'hand over' your patients to the doctor who replaces you. This can usually be done over the phone or a quick coffee. Obviously how much detail you tell your successor depends on whether or not they are familiar with the patients – bear in mind that they may not know them at all. You need to make sure your successors know:

1 Who your patients are, which ward they are on and why they are in hospital.
2 A brief summary of the management of each patient (e.g. awaiting surgery tomorrow, NBM, needs continuous morphine infusion for pain relief but stable).
3 Likely complications or difficulties and how you have been dealing with these to date.
4 Anyone (doctor/nurse/relatives) who may be contacted if problems arise.
5 If you are handing over to a locum who is new to the hospital, you will help him or her enormously by spending a few minutes giving him or her key information about the lay-out of the hospital and how to perform routine tasks (see Locums, p. 199).

Hand backs

It is common to 'hand back' patients to consultants who have looked after them within the last 1–2 years, but check your hospital's policy. It is helpful to hand back patients as early in the day as possible to give the accepting team a fair chance to assess the patient themselves. It is good practice to make sure that investigations suggested on the post-take round have been completed prior to the hand back. The accepting doctor should be aware of any outstanding tests, and the admitting team's provisional diagnosis. Don't forget to explain to the patient what is happening!

Referral letters

If you need to refer a patient to another team, you can either phone the registrar of that team and leave relevant details in the patient's notes, or write the consultant a letter, or both. If you write a letter, include the following:

1 Address the letter to the consultant of the other team.
2 Name of your consultant, yourself and your bleep number.
3 Name of patient, age, sex, DOB, hospital ID and current location (e.g. ward/home).
4 Name of patient's GP.
5 Specific question(s) your team needs answered.
6 Relevant clinical history and examination findings.
7 Recent investigations (including negatives).
8 When you need his or her advice by.
• Try to anticipate which investigations

the other team might need, and have them ready. For example, surgeons almost always need a recent FBC and maybe ECG if they are considering theatre. Gastroenterologists, or any specialist doing a biopsy, will want an INR if investigating liver complaints. See pp. 120–125 for a list of investigations that different specialists are likely to need.

Self-discharge

However it may feel, hospitals are not prisons. Unless patients are likely to incur life-threatening harm to themselves, you cannot restrain them from leaving hospital (even when it is patently idiotic for them to do so). If your patient does decide to leave against your advice, try the following:

• Explain to them why they should stay.
• Inform your senior.
• Have the patient sign a self-discharge note. This is usually available from the ward clerk. If necessary, you can write one yourself. It is a good idea to have a second witness to sign the note:

I, (*Jo Bloggs*) hereby state that I am leaving (*Name of Hospital*) against medical advice on (*today's date*). Witnessed by Dr (*Your surname*), (*today's date*) and (*Colleague's name, today's date*)

    (Jo Blogg's signature)
    (Your name and signature)
    (Second witness name and
     signature)

• Rarely, you may consider using the Mental Health Act to section a patient and restrain them from leaving. Always seek senior advice before doing this (p. 208).
• Make a brief note of what happened in the patient's notes.
• Inform the patient's GP that the patient has self-discharged.

Sick notes

You may be asked to write a sick note for patients to verify that they have been unable to work. There are two types of sick notes you can write:

1 If the patient is *not* trying to claim state benefit, they need a hand-written note on hospital-headed paper. The easiest way to address it is 'To Whom It May Concern' along the top, followed by something like: 'Mrs A has been an inpatient at the X Hospital from 24–30 April and will be unable to return to work until May 7.' Sign and date it, and block print your name and position under your signature as well as the name of the patient's consultant.

  • In this kind of letter, you should *not* disclose the patient's condition. If in doubt, ask your senior.

2 If the patient *is* trying to claim state benefit after leaving hospital, they need a **Med 3** form to be signed by you (ask your ward clerk, registrar or phone the nearest DSS office). This is self-explanatory, but you must fill in the diagnosis. Ask your senior if you have any doubts about it.

Chapter 4: Accident and emergency

Working shifts in A&E can be a lot of fun, or it can result in the weekend from hell, working 'til you drop. As usual, being organized and armed with a few hints makes a big difference to coping well.

General

During both medical and surgical takes you see the same handful of conditions most of the time (see below). Whatever your baseline knowledge, you soon become adept at treating them.
• Do not be afraid to ask nurses for advice. They have seen it all before.
• You can spend a lot of time looking for equipment in casualty. Try preparing batches of forms and bottles when things are quiet. Suggested forms include (per patient):
  2 history sheets, drug chart, fluid chart, X-ray form, blood cards, consent form.
• Try equipping yourself with a metal trolley at the beginning of the shift. It helps to keep your equipment in one place and gives you a surface to work on.
• Try sticking a yellow plastic bag to the edge of the trolley for rubbish; it saves trips to the garbage with packaging. A small yellow sharps bin is ideal if you can find one. Otherwise use a papier-mache kidney dish for sharps and empty it into the sharps bin when it's full.
• Dehydration is a real problem if you

work without a break in casualty. Suggest to the medical or surgical hospital manager that a drinking water dispenser be installed in casualty. Drink as many fluids as you can
• Take meal breaks ruthlessly. Hold the fort for your colleagues and have them do the same for you. No-one works efficiently with hypoglycaemia.
• It is easier to move in casualty without a white coat. This is possible even if you wear a pocketless skirt; clip pens and bleep to your waistband. Alternatively wear a travel pouch.

Admitting and allocating patients

1 Ask medical and nursing colleagues about the local routine for admitting and allocating patients during take.
2 When a GP telephones you to admit a patient:
  • Be polite.
  • Have paper and pen ready.
  • Listen first.
  • Take down: Name.
             Age.
             Problem.
             Hospital number.
             GP name and
               number.
             When to expect the
               patient's arrival.
  • Phone casualty or the ward with the patient's details.
  • Let your senior know that the pa-

tient is coming in and their main complaint.

3 If you accept a patient from a GP, you are obliged to clerk them, even if it is obvious that they need to be transferred to another specialty. Therefore try to transfer the call to the right specialist *before* the patient arrives, or you will end up seeing the patient, however inappropriately.

4 You may bear the brunt of poor bed allocation. Consider negotiating with admissions, the managing sister or charge nurse ('bed manager') and clinical managers to work out a better system. It helps to know the wards' bed status when working in A&E, so you can send patients where you want them.

Keeping track of patients

• Whatever you do, get results for patients before you go to bed, and make sure you have them ready for the post-take ward round.

• Try keeping a history sheet with patient stickers down one side, with results of baseline tests and a thumbnail sketch of the patient next to each sticker. This is invaluable for post-take ward rounds.

• If you are missing results, check the casualty result book before retiring.

• If you urgently need a result after midnight, you can usually get recent results from the technician's book in the lab. There is usually a duty biochemist or haematologist on call.

Medicine

On admission, try to complete for each medical patient:

1 History and examination.
2 Baseline tests: FBC, C&E, glucose, ESR, CRP
MSU and dipstick
ECG
CXR (consider erect CXR if suspected perforation)
Consider clotting screen (INR/ KCCT), LFTs
3 IV access.
4 Fluid chart for 24 hours.
5 Drug chart.

The most common medical emergencies

1 Haematemesis (peptic ulcer or gastritis)
2 Unstable angina
3 MI
4 Stroke (infarct or haemorrhagic)
5 DVT and PE
6 'Off legs' or collapse
7 Overdose

Overdose

Medical House Officers see many patients who have overdosed. A&E get the slashed wrists and other forms of bodily mutilation, but you have to deal with people's gastric contents. Do not panic with overdose patients. There is usually more time than you realize to sort them out, and the vast majority do not take devastating overdoses. You can (and should) get senior medical and nursing assistance if the patient *is* in a critical condition. They may need transfer to ITU. Never wash out an uncooperative or unconscious patient without the supervision of an anaesthetist.

In general

• If in **any** doubt about how to treat someone, phone the 24-hour Poisons hotline (switchboard and A&E staff will have these numbers). Their staff will tell you exactly what to do, according to your patient's symptoms and history.

Poisons information	
Belfast	01232-240 503
Birmingham	0121-507 5588
	0121-507 5589
Cardiff	01222-709 901
Dublin	00353-1-837 9964
	00353-1-837 9966
Edinburgh	0131-536 2300
Leeds	0113-243 0715
London	0171-635 9191
	0171-955 5095
Newcastle	0191-232 5131

• The *BNF* has an excellent section on treatments for different substance overdoses at the beginning of the book (look under 'Poison' in the index). We have not tried to replicate the *BNF* information here, as it is more detailed and up to date in the *BNF* itself.

Treating the patient:

First, briefly assess the patient

1 If the patient is unconscious, seek senior help. Make sure the unconscious patient is in the coma position and check the airway for tongue, dentures or vomit.
2 If the patient is drowsy or unconscious, alert an anaesthetist to intubate the patient for a washout. Get senior advice. The patient may need to be transferred to ITU.

3 Quickly check for and treat hypoxia, hypotension and hypovolaemia (from vomiting and tachypnoea), hypoglycaemia, hypothermia and arrhythmias. Ask the nurses to do a blood glucose stick, ECG, BP and pulse oximeter reading, particularly if the patient is semi-conscious. Consider doing a blood gas and rectal temperature.
4 Secure IV access. Consider immediate, rapid IV fluid if the patient is in shock.
5 Take the following samples from the patient:
  Biochemistry sample
    C&E, urea, salicylate and paracetamol levels. These need repeating if less than 4 hours have elapsed since the overdose
  Glucose sample
    (liver damage causes hypoglycaemia)
  Serum sample (at least one)
    Storage – in case there is need to do further tests
  Sample of vomitus (to biochemistry)
    Label with time, date and suspected substance
It is standard practice to check drug levels (principally salicylate and paracetamol) for all overdose patients. Patients may conceal or simply not realize how many tablets they have taken, or whether they contain these substances. Paracetamol levels should be taken not less than 4 hours after ingestion, aspirin not less than 6 hours, but longer if the tables have enteric coating.
• Always collect at least one sample of blood from the patient, regardless of what they claim to have taken.
• Lethal paracetamol overdoses may not become apparent for several days, when the person starts to go yellow.

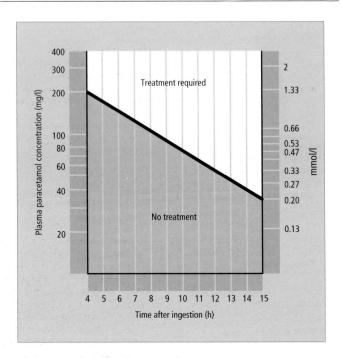

Fig 4.1 Chart to decide who should receive Parvolex.

Always assume that the person has taken paracetamol, and more than they say they have. The *Parvolex* treatment chart found in A&E (see Fig. 4.1) is used to assess whether or not the patient needs treatment with a *Parvolex* infusion (acetylcysteine—see the *BNF* for dosage) to counteract a paracetamol overdose. Take blood levels at least 4 hours (but less than 8) after the patient has ingested the tablets.

If the level is *on or above* the line, the patient needs urgent treatment or risks fatal liver damage. Be prepared for potentially serious side effects, including bronchospasm, hypoglycaemia, shock and vomiting. Glucose should be checked hourly.

Levels *below* the line do not require treatment at present unless the patient has existing liver damage or is taking enzyme-inducing drugs such as carbamazepine. Consult with your senior. Levels need to be re-checked to make sure that they are not rising.

• Aspirin overdose causes metabolic acidosis, therefore consider doing arterial blood gases. Symptoms and signs include tachypnoea, tachycardia and tinnitus.

Second, decide if the patient needs to be washed out or treated with ipecacuanha (Ipecac)

Washouts

NEVER wash out an unconscious patient without first intubating the patient with an anaesthetist's assistance. Usually you should wash patients out within:

4 hours for anything **except corrosive agents and petrol**.

6 hours for opiates and anticholinergics.

12 hours for salicylates, aminophylline, tricyclic antidepressants.

• Washouts are more effective than *Ipecac*.

• Ask someone to show you how to do your first few washouts. Believe it or not, you will soon get used to it!

• Gum boots and a plastic apron save your clothes during washouts.

• Be sure to use *warm* water to wash the patient out. Cold water is painful and may induce angina.

• Coat the hose-pipe with lubricant jelly before insertion; it makes it much easier to swallow.

• Don't forget to follow the water washout with a bottle of charcoal solution to prevent further absorption.

• Save a specimen jar of vomitus for biochemical analysis.

Ipecac

• Give the patient 30 ml of Ipecac followed by a glass of water. Repeat after 20 minutes if necessary. As the patient starts to retch, ensure that they drink water or squash (1–3 jugfuls if possible).

• After the patient has finished vomiting, give them charcoal solution to drink. Put it in a china mug rather than a glass.

• Send a specimen jar of vomitus for biochemical analysis.

Patients refusing treatment

• You *can* section someone who refuses to be treated (see p. 208) if you think they have taken something that may be lethal. Obviously use this as a last resort. Sectioning someone is a complex process and may have serious consequences for them. Get senior advice. Sometimes when faced with the prospect of being sectioned, patients change their mind about being washed out.

Third, do a more thorough history and examination

1 If possible, get a thorough history from the patient *as well as* from whoever accompanied them to hospital. If possible, try to ascertain:

A What precipitated the attempt?

• Intention at time of overdose (did they mean to kill themselves?)

• Previous intentions (have they felt like this often?)

• Was the attempt impulsive or premeditated?

• Did they try to avoid being found?

• Did they leave a note?

• Did the patient take illicit drugs or alcohol?
• Did the patient have specific problems that caused them to consider suicide?
B How likely are they to try to kill themselves again?
• How do they feel about being alive?
• Do they still want to die?
• Psychiatric disorder, especially depressive disorders with insomnia, anorexia and weight loss
• Chronic/serious physical disorder
• Alcohol dependence
• Social isolation
• Unemployment
• Male
• >50 years old
2 Examine the patient thoroughly.
3 Perform a mini-mental test score (see p. 209).

Fourth, discuss the patient with your senior if you haven't already. You will probably need to refer the patient to the psychiatrists

Surgery

On admission, try to complete:
1 History and examination.
2 Baseline tests: FBC, C&E, glucose, amylase, G&S or cross-match
MSU & dipstick, consider pregnancy test
ECG
AXR, consider erect CXR

3 IV access.
4 Fluid chart for 24 hours.
5 Consent.
6 Drug chart.
• It is cruel to leave patients in acute pain. Ambulance staff and nurses cannot give pain relief until a doctor has seen them. If someone has renal colic, for example, you may be able to ascertain this quickly and prescribe analgesia accordingly.
• Diclofenac sodium (Voltarol) provides effective pain relief for renal colic. It can be given IM or by suppository.
• Very occasionally, patients who are seeking opiates *or* a stay in hospital may fake surgical conditions. Look for needle marks, small pupils and odd histories. If you suspect a patient is faking pain, ask for senior advice. It is extremely dodgy to 'punish' addict patients (or anyone else) with inadequate pain relief. If your patient is an opiate addict *and* has a real surgical condition, then they will need extra relief for severe pain.

Most common conditions for surgical emergency admissions
1 Acute abdomen (appendicitis and other RIF pain, UTI, obstruction, IBD, IBS)
• Always be aware of the possibility of pregnancy or gynaecological conditions in young women with abdominal pain. It is routine to request pregnancy tests on urine specimens
2 Renal colic
3 Changing catheters
• Urological conditions, such as changing catheters, renal colic, haematuria, can sometimes be referred to the urologists

Chapter 5: Becoming a better doctor

Post-graduate medical education used to be fairly limited, to the detriment of doctors' morale and brain cells. Fortunately, 'Continuing Medical Education' is rapidly improving through the post-graduate colleges. There are many things you can do to keep your work interesting and to prevent the whisky bottle from becoming too attractive.

Computers (If you are already a PC hack, skip this section!)

We recommend becoming as computer literate as possible, because so much medical information and worldwide communication is becoming available through the Internet (see below). If it's any consolation, our nearest and dearest relatives who recently shrieked in horror at the thought of booting a disk drive are now happily e-mailing each other over the Internet and doing their accounts using home PCs.

Hardware (i.e. the computer itself): what to buy?

Computer prices are falling rapidly. If you can afford it, it is probably advisable to buy a more advanced machine that you will be happy with for several years and which will keep up with increasingly sophisticated software. We strongly recommend consulting a recent computing magazine for articles that compare different brands and models.

• At the time this book was published, a decent personal computer (either laptop or desk-top model) is a 133 MHz or faster Pentium with 16 Mb RAM, and at least 1.2 Mb HDD (Hard Disk Drive) memory. As databases and journals are increasingly going on-line and becoming available on CD-ROM, it is probably a good idea to buy a package that includes an internal or external **modem** (at least 14.4 bps speed, preferably 28.8 bps), and a good **CD-ROM drive**. The speed of the modem is the main rate limiting step when requesting Internet downloads, particularly when using Internet interface software, such as *Netscape* or *Mosaic*. The **video card memory**, which controls the speed at which images are transferred from the software onto the screen, comes in either 'VRAM' or 'DRAM'; VRAM is superior, but only makes a difference when using animated programs. The usual amount supplied is 1 Mb, although two or more is better. You also need at least 256Kb 'cache space' which enables several programs to run at once (or to 'multi-task') quickly.

• The powerful 'PowerMac' *Apple Macintosh* computers are now relatively price-competitive with the major PC brands, for similar computing power, although PC clones are usually cheaper. Similar specifications for *Apple* computers apply. The *PowerMac* models can translate and use most PC software.

• Make sure that you have a good service and parts warranty for your computer. Ideally, the company will supply an 'on-site' service and parts warranty, which means that it will send a representative to your home for a specified period of time, free of charge, if anything goes wrong.

• Check which software packages come with the computer. Some deals include tons of great software, including full word processing, spreadsheet and graphics programs. You will pay a lot if you have to buy all this yourself.

• When ordering your computer, check the available date of delivery. If you have to wait 3 months, switch firms!

• One good way to buy a computer is to order it directly from the manufacturer, rather than going through a retailer. The (usually toll-free) numbers of companies can be found in the *Yellow Pages* and in any major computing magazine.

• Apparently the P6 computers (which will supersede Pentiums) are at present not much faster than Pentiums; most magazines suggest that Pentiums will remain a good investment for several years.

• Find out from your consultant or BMA office if there is any way you can claim an educational discount (or if the health authority could help you pay for the computer) on the grounds that it helps you with NHS work. Consider claiming it for tax deductibility.

• In addition to magazine consumer surveys, try tracking down the person who maintains and buys computers for your hospital. They may be able to guide you in purchasing a computer.

• Consider buying a lap-top computer, which is much more convenient for the mobile junior doctor. You can always buy a large screen and keyboard to plug into the lap-top if you want to make it easier to use at home.

• If you need to buy a monitor, for enhanced quality of life treat yourself to a 15″ or larger screen (rather than the regular 14″ screen). Bear in mind also that your can buy ergonomic keyboards and mice that can really improve your comfort level if you use the computer a lot.

Software

There are so many different brands of software with a myriad of functions. We suggest that you consider the following generic types of software programs to help organize your files and save you oodles of time while making your work look professional.

1 Word processing package (e.g. Microsoft Word, WordPerfect. It is possible to convert *MS Word* files to *WordPerfect* files and vice versa so it is really a matter of institutional preference which you use. MS Word is probably more widely used within medicine).

2 Bibliographic database package (e.g. *Idealist*, *Procite*, *Reference Manager*). These programs are great if you are interested in keeping long-term files or notes on just about anything. Basically, they enable you to write notes and bibliographic references on whatever you want (such as journal articles and talks you've been to) and then recall any text or reference word with a few key strokes. They are a good way of beating the paper tiger into submission.

3 Slide and overhead presentation package (e.g. *Powerpoint*) – enables you

to make professional-looking slides and overheads.

4 Spreadsheet program (e.g. *Excel*, *Lotus*) enables you to do accounts and present tabulated, quantitative data.

5 Communications software (see under Modem below).

6 Desk-top publishing software (e.g. *PageMaker*) enables you to produce professional-looking newsletters/publications.

7 Virus detection software will prevent your files and computer from being 'infected' with destructive computer viruses.

Modems and communications software

Modems are separate, relatively inexpensive hardware items that enable you to connect your computer to the phone line. A modem enables you to dial into local or distant 'networks', or directly access other people's computers and fax machines. You also need a communications software package so that your computer can 'talk to' the modem and use it effectively. This usually comes with the modem.

Other ways of getting access to on-line databases

There are now at least 5 WWW sites offering free access to MEDLINE. We recommend HealthGate (http://www.healthgate.com) as it has a user friendly search engine. In addition, the BMA now offers free access to MEDLINE, if you are a BMA member and you have a modem. It will, however, cost you the phone call to London. Increasingly, hospital and university libraries have on-line databases available if you have a modem. Other useful medical information providers include: CliniWeb (www.ohsu.edu/cliniweb/search.html) Grateful Med (igm.nlm.nih.gov:80/) (US (NIH) based site), Health On the Net Foundation (Swiss-based organisation) (www.hon.ch/) and OMNI (omni.ac.uk/general-info/search.html) (UK based).

A bit about the Internet

Modems are verging on essential, because they enable you to access the Internet and the rapidly expanding world of international information networks. Why is this so important? We (and lots of others) believe that the world is undergoing something of another technological revolution in which rapid information exchange is transforming the way people live and work. Learning how to access this information will keep you from becoming scared of it — and give you an enormous advantage in your work.

The Internet is a vast, sprawling electronic network which extends as far as there are phone lines (or satellites). It was originally set up by the US military to improve communication between international military stations, but since then it has been somewhat swamped by millions of other users world-wide. The Internet enables individuals from every part of the globe to talk to one another via their computers within seconds, and to tap into whatever information sources lie at the end of the millions of lines.

To tap into the Internet you need to be connected to a local 'node'. Tapping in may cost you money, unless you can connect through a hospital or university that has free access to the Internet (some do and some don't—ask your hospital computer person). Several companies will connect you to a node for £5–10 per month. You may have to pay a fee to connect into certain databases, but many are available for nothing.

We won't wax lyrical here about all the things you can access over the 'Net'. There are tons of user-friendly books on this subject in most large book stores. Medical journals are increasingly advertising databases and users' bulletin boards that can be accessed through the Net and the World Wide Web (WWW).

How to access the Internet
1 Buy and install a modem for your computer communications software package (get help with this from your computer store or hospital computer person).
2 Establish with a local university or hospital how to 'dial in' to their Internet node, or subscribe to a local 'server' (company) which will enable you to access the Internet.
3 Buy or borrow a book about the Internet so that you don't miss out on the tons of information highways/ bulletin boards/public information available.

Keeping up with the literature

The information and technology explosion is very real. There are currently over 25 000 biomedical journals in print, and this figure is rising exponentially[1].

[1] Wyatt J. (1991) Uses and sources of medical knowledge. *Lancet* **338**, 1368–1373.

How on earth can you keep up with the literature?

Actually, you can. There are several great ways to keep up to date with stacks of international journals with minimal fuss (we wish we knew about these when we were students):

• Invest in a personal computer and a bibliographic software package (see p. 22). These allow you to make super-quick notes and references of good things you read or hear so that you can access them years from now. Say goodbye to bulging filing cabinets and disorganized papers and build your own personal database which will serve you for talks, presentations and your own interests for the rest of your professional life.

• Adopt a 'problem-based' approach to reading. This means reading whatever you need to answer real questions, rather than blindly scanning journals with minimal retention and maximum boredom (see Evidence-based medicine). You will remember much more of what you read if your patient depends upon it and you'll probably also find it more interesting.

• If you *do* want to scan scientific studies, try reading the *BMJ*'s new, monthly supplement, *Evidence-Based Medicine* that contains critically appraised summaries of the most recent, good quality medical trials articles from a wide range of international journals.

• Read review articles before you read other kinds of studies. Good quality systematic reviews, especially those using meta-analysis, are the most efficient studies to read[2] because they com-

[2] Milne R., Chambers L. (1993) Assessing the scientific quality of review articles. *Journal of Epidemiology and Community Health* **47**, 169–170.

bine the results of many individual studies, adding statistical power and giving you an efficient overview of the topic. The Cochrane Library (CL) contains both the Cochrane Collaboration and NHS Centre for Reviews and Dissemination's databases of systematic reviews, so should be your first port of call if you have access to them. The CL is currently being installed on hospital computers throughout the UK.

• Did you know that the BMA offers a CD-ROM database of health-related newspaper cuttings? If you need information about something that was in the press, call the BMA on 0171-387 4499.

• Learn how to do critical appraisal on what you read so that you can evaluate studies yourself, rather than relying on the authors' conclusions. It is little known that most published studies, even in leading medical journals, do not have reliable results because the study methodology was not rigorous enough. Critical appraisal is a simple process that enables you to be much more discriminating in what you read (see below in Evidence-based medicine).

Evidence-based medicine

Evidence-based medicine is being introduced into teaching hospitals around the country as this book goes to print. Basically, evidence-based medicine involves using research findings to give clinicians much more statistical power in interpreting every-day clinical data, rather than relying on anecdotal evidence. It may not sound like much, but most people find that evidence-based medicine markedly improves the way they practise medicine.

The idea of evidence-based medicine is not new. People have been using 'the literature' for years to improve clinical decision-making. However, the advent of big, electronic databases such as MEDLINE and the CL (see above) now mean that doctors can rapidly search and evaluate the literature on a regular and systematic basis, especially if these databases are installed on ward and library computers.

Not only do people who practise evidence-based medicine find that they become more aware—and critical—of research findings, but they quickly become adept at solving difficult problems and find they can engage better in medical debates. Evidence-based medicine can be practised by teams or by individuals. Find out about it and try it out!

What does evidence-based medicine involve?

Evidence-based medicine involves carrying out three key steps:

1 Ask a clear question about the problem you are trying to solve (e.g. Should I anticoagulate an elderly woman with asymptomatic atrial fibrillation?).

2 Search the literature for good quality evidence using a structured, hierarchical search that gives you the most statistically powerful research first. Stop when you have enough information to answer your question. Search first for systematic reviews, second for randomized controlled trials, and lastly for other types of studies. To do this efficiently you need access to an electronic database such as the CL and MEDLINE. See your hospital librarian or tap into them

through the BMA or server if you have a computer and modem.

3 Critically appraise (or evaluate) the evidence you have found to see whether or not its findings are reliable and relevant to your situation. To do this you need a list of questions which help you to assess the methodology of the research. These questions are available in: Oxman A.D., Sackett D.L., Guyatt G.H. Users Guides to the Literature I–III, *Journal of the American Medical Association* (1993) **207**, 2093; (1994) **271**, 59; (1994) **271**, 389.

These simple guides take you through the steps of critical appraisal for different kinds of research evidence.

To get to grips with evidence-based practice and critical appraisal, a user-friendly, inexpensive reference manual is: Sackett D.L., Haynes R.B., Guyatt G.H., Tugwell P. (1991) *Clinical Epidemiology. A Basic Science for Clinical Medicine.* 2nd edn. Little, Brown and Company, Toronto. It teaches you how to critically appraise different kinds of evidence including reviews, economic analyses and research about quality of care, therapy, diagnosis, screening, prognosis and disease causation.

Professionalism

No-one teaches you how to be a professional. Don't worry if the transition from student to doctor is full of bumps and jolts—it certainly was for us! There isn't much mystery to being 'professional'; it's mostly about communicating well, building relationships and being responsible for what you say and do. However, this is no small thing to accomplish.

Communication

For an enjoyable house job, good communication is essential. As a House Officer, you will make about 30 phone calls for every patient you admit. You may interview up to 5000 people during the year. You will write volumes of notes that others will rely on and that might one day be used as evidence in court. You will physically touch hundreds of people.

Unfortunately, many medical schools do not teach communication or relationship skills: you are supposed to pick them up from your seniors. As you have probably already observed, many seniors are singularly lacking in personal and communication skills. It pays to develop your own skills; they will save you bleeps, headaches, time, and law suits. Over 90% of UK medical defence cases result from poor communication rather than from negligence *per se*. Most so-called ward 'personality clashes' can be solved by effective and imaginative communication.

1 It is really important and very difficult to write legibly at 3 am. If you are right-handed, try using a fountain pen—it's harder to scrawl with.

2 Write your name and bleep number on ward boards. This is very helpful for the nursing staff if you are on call (e.g. 14 May cover: Jo Bloggs' bleep 1413).

3 Let people know if you are very distressed about something. Try not to transform grief or fatigue into defensive behaviour, such as silence or arrogance. People are usually pretty good at helping you out if they know what's up.

4 ESP is not a reliable form of commu-

nication; short notes and phone calls work much better.

5 Most junior doctors lose their heads from time to time. Don't be afraid to say you're sorry. People usually respect apologies.

6 If conflicts arise, some useful tips include[3]:

- Ask yourself, are you sure you're right?
- Does it matter?
- Try turning difficult questions back to the patient. For example, you can ask them: 'What makes you ask that question?'[4]
- Try to appear calm, despite what you may feel inside.

7 People around the country have made video tapes to help people understand choices about treatments more thoroughly. Contact a lecturer nurse, librarian or district health authority to find out if any are readily available.

8 Use an interpreter if necessary. Interpreters can usually be contacted through the switch board or the casualty nursing staff.

Consultants and senior registrars

- Each consultant will have about five things that they want to know about each patient (sometimes for no apparent reason). Find these out early and supply them tirelessly, no matter what they are.

[3] Hope R.A. *et al.* (1994). *Oxford Practice Skills Project: sample teaching materials*. Oxford Medical School, Oxford.
[4] Macguire P., Faulkner A. (1988) Communicate with cancer patients: Handling bad news and difficult questions. *British Medical Journal* **297**, 970–974.

Your predecessor is usually a good source of this kind of information.

- NEVER say you've done something when you haven't.
- Impress your seniors by being straightforward and by knowing your patients well. This matters much more in your house job than having read the latest *NEJM*.

GPs

You will talk and write to many GPs; some you will get to know quite well. The following are some recommendations from Joe Rosenthal, a GP who also teaches at the Royal Free Hospital in London:

1 Phone requests for admission:

- Have paper and pen ready.
- Be polite.
- Listen first.
- Take down: Name
             Age
             Problem
             Hospital number
             GP name and
                number
             Expected time of
                admission.
- Inform casualty.

2 Phone the GP on discharge if the patient:

- Self-discharges.
- Is in an unstable condition.
- Has poor home circumstances.
- Dies.
- Needs an early visit.

3 Discharge letter

Complete before the patient leaves! Include:

- Patient details.
- Name of consultant.
- Name of ward.

- Diagnosis and important negative findings.
- Treatment given.
- Treatment on discharge.
- Follow-up arrangements.
- What the patient has been told.
- Your name and bleep number.

Nurses

It is pretty crucial to get on with nurses, who are fantastic allies. They know most of what you need to know as an House Officer and are usually keen and willing to teaching you. Nurses are trained in a range of things that doctors aren't and vice versa, so the teams are complementary–use this to your advantage! Here are some hints for starters:

- Always introduce yourself to nurses and other staff when you're new on a ward.
- Always tidy up after yourself. Especially tidy up your own sharps. Most needlestick injuries arise from sharps someone else left hidden.
- Tidy up your trolley after any procedure. Find out in the first couple of weeks how to make up your own trolley and how to pack it away.
- Don't expect nurses to do things they are not qualified to do. Nurses may have extended roles (such as IV drug administration) but they may not. Nurses can be struck off much more easily than doctors.
- Do unto nurses as they do to you. Make them cups of tea or coffee or offer to do an IV round if you're on the ward without much to do. This helps to create an easy, generous atmosphere on the ward which makes coming to work much more fun.

- To avoid heaps of bleeps, ask nurses to write down tasks and have one nurse bleep you with the list every couple of hours or so. Tell them you will return to do a round at a specific time.
- If multiple bleeps are a real problem, consider arranging a meeting with the medical or surgical manager and nursing staff to work out a better system. This is the sort of thing hospital managers are employed for. Talk to your senior if s/he is supportive.
- If you have a plan in your head for a patient, or can foresee a problem a patient might have (e.g. a delayed discharge date), let the nursing, social work and occupational therapy staff know so they can help you with it, rather than having to nag you for information.
- Write instructions to nurses in the medical notes.
- Save time: get to know how team nursing works on your ward. Basically, team nursing means that nurses work in independent, often colour-coded teams, each of which looks after a certain number of patients. Do not try to elicit information about a 'red' patient from a 'green' nurse (see below under Team nursing).
- Nurses often work in three 8-hour shifts. Their rota is usually kept in the nurses' office. It is often helpful to know when a particular nurse will be available.
- Try not to interrupt nurses when they are meeting for the shift 'report' and handover.

Helpful things to know about nurses

- Nursing grades (varies between hospitals):
Student nurse:

attends university for 3–4 years (4 years if a degree course).

Staff nurse:

graded D–F (A–C are auxiliary nurses).

Sisters:

graded F–H (usually).

Nurse managers:

graded H–J.

Lecturer practitioner:

senior specialist nurse who teaches and advises more inexperienced staff. Nurse practitioners (extensively used in North America) are gradually increasing in number but are still relatively thin on the ground in the UK.

• Nursing jargon:

Bank nurse is a nurse hired temporarily from a 'bank' agency.

Charge nurse is a male version of ward sister.

Team nursing means that nurses work in colour-coded teams, each of which independently cares for different groups of patients. It means that nurses get to know their patients better. It also means that nurses may not know much about patients who aren't assigned to their team. If you want to know about a 'blue' patient, ask a 'blue-team' nurse.

To 'special' is to provide intensive nursing for a seriously ill patient.

Ward sister is the female version of charge nurse who may have overall responsibility for the patients.

Back/Late shift is the shift from approximately 2 pm to 9 pm.

Early shift is the shift from approximately 7 am to 2 pm.

• Things nurses hate most:

Doctors treating them like second class citizens.

Doctors not answering bleeps reasonably quickly (so they have to wait by the phone for ages).

Doctors leaving sharps (and other rubbish) around.

Doctors not explaining things well to patients and not informing the nurse what they found out from the patient.

Patients (see also p. 85 Breaking bad news)

• Listen to patients, even if you think their worries are trivial. Remember that you don't have to solve all their problems. Just listening can be a huge help.

• If you do not have time to listen to a patient properly, either organize for someone else to listen (such as their nurse) or tell the patient you'll sit down with them later. Preferably give the patient a time and stick to it.

• If you cannot make it back to talk to a patient, phone their nurse to tell the patient so they aren't left waiting.

• Avoid medical jargon when talking to patients (e.g. 'blockage' not 'stenosis').

• Give people information in bite-size chunks which they can manage. This is especially important for people who are anxious or when you're relaying scary information.

• Use conceptually clear diagrams wherever possible to explain yourself, as shown in the Appendix (remember that anatomically correct diagrams may be more confusing than conceptually clear ones).

• Be straight with patients. Answer questions honestly, even if it means saying that you don't know.

• Do not be pushed into committing yourself to a diagnosis if you don't have good evidence for it.

Patients' families

Patients' families often suffer from lack of information from hospital staff. You can greatly alleviate this with minimal effort and you will be showered with gratitude. If possible, take the patient's nurse with you to ensure continuity of care. There are two main problems you can help with:

Information about patient discharge

Making arrangements for home care can be a major ordeal, particularly for families where everyone works. You can make a big difference if you or the nurse can let the family know as soon as possible:

1 When (and if) the patient can go home; if possible, morning or afternoon. It may be possible for your patient to leave at a time that is convenient for family routines.

2 Special instructions that the patient will need to follow at home and when they should go and see their GP.

3 Drugs that will be needed and when in the near future.

4 Who they can contact if something goes wrong.

5 What you have asked the GP to arrange in the near future.

Hints

• Find out the discharge procedure from nurses.

• Be aware of hospital visiting hours so that you can tell families when patients are admitted.

• Liaise with nurses, social workers and occupational therapists, as they often have important information for patients and their families on discharge.

• Remember that many people will not challenge a doctor, but may put up with a lot of hassle to do what you say, even when it makes no difference to the ward. If families are looking bothered, ask them what's wrong. You may be able to help with little effort.

• Imagine the patient was your relative and you had to look after them – what would you need to know?

• Ask family members if they have any questions.

Information about what's wrong with the patient (see p. 85 for Breaking bad news)

Your main duty is to care for the patient, not their family; you should get the patient's permission before divulging information to any family member. Taking time in a non-stressful environment to explain things to family members can be invaluable. Families remember how doctors explained things to them. Key features that we find make a difference include:

• Take the family to a private room. This enables people to remember information and ask questions.

• Try to get rid of your bleep. Hand it to a colleague.

• Have all investigations and findings to hand. Be ready to answer lots of questions and be ready to admit uncertainty.

• Write in the notes what you have told the family and tell the nursing staff.

• Have tissues and cups of tea handy if possible.

• If possible, collect all family members for one chat. Otherwise they turn up at all sorts of times and you have to repeat yourself.

Confidentiality

Breaches of confidentiality may be both unlawful and amount to professional misconduct, and you may be called upon to justify any such breach. Keeping confidentiality is not always as easy as it sounds – you may need to discuss patient histories with many people, both within the hospital and the community. The following guidelines should help you to keep legal confidentiality:

• Refer to patients by name as little as possible.
• Do not discuss confidential information with people over the phone unless you are certain of their identity, and that they are authorized to receive the information.
• Never discuss patients in public places, such as lifts and hospital canteens.
• *Never* discuss anything with the press if approached. Refer immediately to your consultant or the hospital manager.
• Refer police officers to your senior.
• Take care when discussing patients over the phone. Transfer ward calls to the doctors' office wherever possible. It is easy to find yourself shouting above the noise of a ward only to find that the entire ward can hear you.
• Remember that curtains are not sound proof. If you have confidential or delicate information to convey or obtain,

consider taking the patient to a side room.
• Do not talk about patients so that they may be identified outside of immediately relevant hospital settings. For example, don't tell your dinner guests stories about patients that they may recognize, even if you don't name them. It is better to avoid this kind of thing altogether, however entertaining it may be.
• The MDU and MPS both have 24-hour advice lines if you are a member.

Exceptions to keeping confidentiality

There are common sense exceptions to confidentiality, such as when you have good reason to believe that the patient is likely to cause death or serious harm to him or herself or others. Sometimes it may not be clear cut as to whether you should or shouldn't respect confidentiality. For example, if a patient admits a crime to you, should you tell anyone about it? Whichever is the case:

• Always ask your consultant for advice.
• Document your decision and other relevant information in the notes to cover yourself in the event of a court case, or complaint. Your medical defense insurer can advise you if you are in any doubt.

Consent See p. 181.

Chapter 6: Cardiac arrests and crash calls

You will almost certainly be a junior member of the hospital crash team. If you are first on the scene, the absolute priority is to ensure adequate ventilation and perfusion—basic life support. It is one occasion when a well learnt plan of action is essential.

You do not have time to 'make a diagnosis'. Stay calm and then:

1 Make sure the airway is clear and secured and that someone (preferably two people working in rotations) is doing adequate CPR. Help if necessary.

2 Secure IV access if basic life support is already being provided and there is a 'spare pair of hands' but do not waste time if you are struggling to put in an IV line. Get help fast and do point 3 in the meanwhile.

3 Get an ECG trace. If there is no chest lead monitor, this is quickly done by placing the defibrillator paddles over the chest.

Decide on a course of action according to the algorithm (Fig. 6.1); based on the new Advanced Life Support (ALS) guidelines (Resuscitation Council (UK) 1997). We strongly recommend you read the guidelines in full (available from the ALS course coordinator in your hospital).

Hints

1 Find out on day one of your job how the defibrillator works and learn the layout of your hospital's arrest trolley. Get on an advanced life support (ALS) course as soon as possible.

2 Note the time of the crash call so you can keep track of how long the resuscitation has been in progress.

3 Go to bed dressed in surgical scrubs if you are carrying the crash bleep. Time does matter and should not be wasted getting 'properly' dressed.

4 It is useful to know the patient's medical background although this is not a priority. Especially look for risk factors of:

- Exsanguinating bleed (e.g. oesophageal varices, recent surgery, bleeding disorder).
- Pneumothorax (e.g. recent central line placement, surgical procedures).
- Pericardial tamponade (e.g. recent chest trauma, recent MI).
- Pulmonary embolus (e.g. recent DVT, major pelvic surgery).
- MI (e.g. history of IHD).
- Electrolyte imbalance, especially $K+$ levels (e.g. anuric patient after major sugery, patient with severe renal impairment).

5 Cardiac arrest is traumatic for other patients on the ward. Use professional language and stay calm.

6 After an unsuccessful call, be sensitive to the fact that nurses and other doctors may have had a close relationship with the patient.

7 It is always worth checking that the patient is not 'not for resus in the event of cardiac arrest'. This should always be written clearly in the notes When in doubt your duty is to attempt to save the patient's life.

Unresponsive

Are you alright?

No breathing

No pulse

Open airway

AIRWAY

Rescue breathing

BREATHING

CPR

CIRCULATION

2:15

Call for help

Including:
- defibrillator
- airway adjuncts
- oxygen
- emergency kit

Consider

- precordial thump in witnessed or monitored arrest

- 2 Rescuer CPR

1:5

- and mouth-to-mask ventilation

Fig. 6.1 Protocol for the treatment of cardiac arrest cases in hospitals. From leaflet produced by Leardal Medical Ltd and The Resuscitation Council (UK).

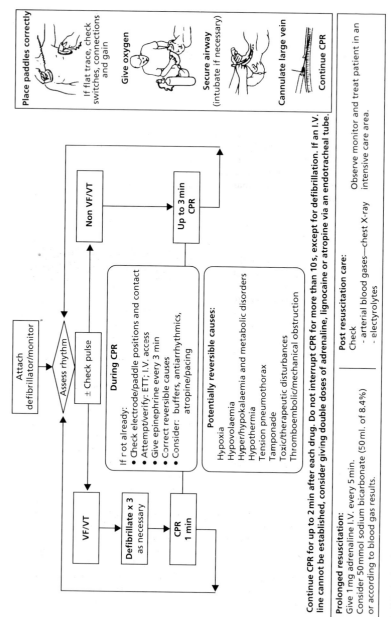

Place paddles correctly

If flat trace, check switches, connections and gain

Give oxygen

Secure airway (intubate if necessary)

Cannulate large vein

Continue CPR

Attach defibrillator/monitor

Assess rhythm

± Check pulse

VF/VT

Non VF/VT

Defibrillate x 3 as necessary

CPR 1 min

Up to 3 min CPR

During CPR

If not already:
- Check electrode/paddle positions and contact
- Attempt/verify: ETT; I.V. access
- Give epinephrine every 3 min
- Correct reversible causes
- Consider: buffers, antiarrhythmics, atropine/pacing

Potentially reversible causes:

Hypoxia
Hypovolaemia
Hyper/hypokalaemia and metabolic disorders
Hypothermia
Tension pneumothorax
Tamponade
Toxic/therapeutic disturbances
Thromboembolic/mechanical obstruction

Continue CPR for up to 2 min after each drug. Do not interrupt CPR for more than 10s, except for defibrillation. If an I.V. line cannot be established, consider giving double doses of adrenaline, lignocaine or atropine via an endotracheal tube.

Prolonged resuscitation:
Give 1 mg adrenaline I.V. every 5 min.
Consider 50 mmol sodium bicarbonate (50 ml. of 8.4%) or according to blood gas results.

Post resuscitation care:
Check
- arterial blood gases—chest X-ray
- electrolytes

Observe monitor and treat patient in an intensive care area.

Fig. 6.1 Continued

Chapter 7: Common calls

This section provides help with problems you are likely to get bleeped for. In particular, it helps you to exclude serious conditions and to initiate mainstay management.

How to use this section

Like a recipe book, this section lists basic protocols for common calls. We recommend the following:
• When first using the chapter, read the short blurb immediately beneath each call, which lists the most likely causes of each problem and things to watch out for. Differential diagnoses are listed in the way that makes them easiest to remember. Most of the time, this is in order of likelihood in the hospital setting.
• Feel free to scribble in the margins and make modifications to each 'recipe' in light of the clinical context and seniors' preferences. You probably will not need to carry out each step for every patient.
• To make this section easy to use in the middle of the night, we have kept abbreviations to a minimum. If in doubt, please refer to the abbreviations index (p. xiv). Drug abbreviations are as follows:

od	once in 24 hours
bd	twice in 24 hours
tds	three times in 24 hours
qds	four times in 24 hours
PO	orally
SC	subcutaneously
IM	intramuscularly
IV	intravenously
nocte	at night
mane	in the morning
stat	straight away
ī, īī	one tablet, two tablets

Considerations for all ward calls

• Never hesitate to call your seniors. It is their job to back you up.
• Always examine patients in a good light even if it means switching on the main lights.
• Even in dire emergencies, act steadily and reassure the patient.
• The key to managing simultaneous bleeps is to prioritize tasks according to urgency and location in the hospital.
• Keep emergency routines fresh in your mind throughout the year. Patients can deteriorate when you least expect it, such as on convalescent wards.
• Before going to bed, check that you know where to find: ophthalmoscope/ otoscope; stethoscope; patella hammer; blood-taking equipment; catheter sets; blood gas machines; ECG machine; and blood fridges.
• While on call, wear respectable pyjamas such as theatre scrubs.
• If you are tired or woken from a deep sleep, try washing your face in cold water and mentally preparing yourself for

the problem you are about to deal with. Consider differential diagnoses as you walk to the ward.
• After seeing patients, sit down with their notes and review their history to make sure you haven't missed something, and document your findings.
• Whatever you are called for, don't forget to check the fluid and drug charts.
• When tired, try not to argue with nursing or medical colleagues. If you feel you are being bleeped unnecessarily, take the matter up when you are well rested.
• Don't be too hard on yourself if everything seems daunting. It is! Experience is the only way to develop good clinical judgement and familiarity with practical procedures.

Abdominal pain

Your priority is to exclude peritonism and obstruction. Common causes of non-acute abdominal pain, such as UTI, constipation and post-op pain, are not life threatening but may require treatment.

When answering your bleep, ask for

• BP, pulse and T.
• Dipstick urine for protein and blood.
• Keep the patient NBM.

Differential diagnoses
Intestinal obstruction
• Constipation
• Adhesions
• Hernia, volvulus, tumour

Peritonism
• Inflammation or infection of any intra-abdominal organ: pancre-atitis, cholecystitis, appendicitis, diverticulitis
• Perforated viscus
• Complications of pregnancy
• Gynaecological causes (ovarian) torsion etc.)
• Leaking abdominal aortic aneurysm
• Intestinal infarction

Peptic ulceration/gastritis

Extra-peritoneal causes
• Urinary retention
• UTI
• Wound abscess
• Basal pneumonia
• Inferior MI (often with associated N&V)
• Retro-peritoneal bleed or abscess
• DKA

On the ward

1 See the patient immediately. If flat, call for senior help and commence basic life support. See The moribund patient, p. 70.
2 If the patient is stable, take a more thorough history and examine the patient. Don't forget to consider:
• Medical history: alcohol, diabetes, IBD, IHD, recent procedures, previous surgery, and shingles.
• Pain—localization and radiation, onset, character, relieving/aggravating factors, associated symptoms.
• LMP.
• PR and FOB.
• Extra-abdominal causes.
• Exclude *peritonism*: localized or generalized peritonitis: fever, guarding, rebound tenderness, absent bowel sounds.
• Exclude *obstruction*: no flatus, no

bowel motion, vomiting, cramping abdominal pain and abdominal distension. Check hernial orifices.

3 Investigations to consider:
  • FBC and INR.
  • C&E, urea, Ca, amylase and glucose.
  • G&S.
  • ABGs if acutely unwell, or if you suspect pancreatitis or intestinal ischaemia.
  • Radiology: erect CXR (free air under diaphragm, pneumonia), supine/erect AXR (check for air–fluid levels, intestinal distension, calcifications, air in biliary tree).
  • ECG to rule out MI.
  • MSU for UTI (a common cause of abdominal pain in hospital) and urinary dipstick for blood or protein.

Hints

• Don't delay analgesia once you have examined the abdomen.
• Involve the surgical team early if necessary.
• Gastritis and non-perforating peptic ulcers can cause severe epigastric pain but not true peritonism. The pain is usually relieved within minutes by antacids.
• Free air under the diaphragm may persist for more than a week after abdominal surgery or laparoscopy.

Anaemia

You will usually be called by the lab for gross anaemia. In this case, your immediate concerns are to exclude bleeding and heart failure. Chronic anaemia should always be investigated before transfusion unless the Hb is below 6 g/dl (see Table 7.1). By far the commonest cause of anaemia is occult blood loss.

On the ward

1 See the patient and assess the need for transfusion. Try to avoid transfusion until the diagnosis is clear, unless:
  • Hb is dangerously low (<6 g/dl).
  • Patient is overtly symptomatic (feeling faint, SOB at rest, tachycardia, angina, postural hypotension or has had serious acute blood loss).
Where possible, avoid transfusions in patients with:
  • Haemoglobinopathies, especially thalassaemia. They can usually cope with low Hbs. Consult with your senior and haematologist.
  • Patients with B_{12} deficiency, as it may precipitate heart failure.

Table 7.1 Differential diagnoses of anaemia.

Low MCV (<76 fl)	Normal MCV (76–96 fl)	High MCV (>96 fl)

Iron deficiency
  Bleeding (GI, vaginal)
  Nutritional
Thalassaemia
Sideroblastic anaemia
	Acute blood loss
	Haemolysis
	Chronic infection or
	  inflammation
	Malignancy
	Pregnancy
	Renal failure
		B_{12} or folate deficiency
		Liver disease
		Alcoholism
		Marrow infiltration
		Hypothyroidism
		Reticulocytosis
		Acquired sideroblastic anaemia

2 Take a history and examine the patient. Don't forget to consider:
  • Occult GI bleeding—dyspepsia, weight loss, change in bowel habit.
  • Menorrhagia.
  • Medication (NSAIDs, drugs causing haemolysis, marrow suppression).
  • Jaundice, skin rashes, lymph nodes.
  • Abdomen: splenomegaly, ascites.
  • PR and FOB.
  • CVS—signs of SBE, prosthetic valves.
  • CNS—signs of peripheral neuropathy or dementia (B_{12} deficiency or alcoholism).
3 Investigations to consider:
  • Repeat FBC.
  • G&S or cross-match.
  • Iron studies, B_{12}, folate, and blood film.
  • C&E, urea, liver function tests.
  • LDH as a useful marker of haemolysis.
  • Other tests (e.g. bone marrow biopsy), according to the differential diagnoses.

Hints

• Iron-deficiency anaemia is not an end diagnosis—you need to investigate its cause. The commonest are occult GI blood loss due to peptic ulcer disease, colonic tumours, menorrhagia, poor diet and pregnancy.
• Be alert to mild anaemia when checking routine blood results. Slight Hb deficits are easy to miss and can be an early sign of serious disease.
• Leukoerythroblastic anaemia means there are primitive red and white cells in the peripheral circulation. The patient may need a bone marrow biopsy and investigation for occult malignancy.

Arrhythmia

While abnormalities in the heart rate and rhythm are relatively common and usually non-life threatening, never be afraid to call the crash team *before* the patient arrests! You are not expected to diagnose and manage arrhythmias without senior advice.

When answering your bleep

Ask nursing staff for pulse, BP and T and to give O_2 if the patient is unwell.

Initial management for all arrhythmias

On the ward

1 See the patient. Check ABC. If flat, have someone call the crash team and commence CPR. Give 100% O_2.
2 If the patient is well and stable, take a brief history and examination. Don't forget to consider:
  • Cardiac symptoms (chest pain, palpitations, breathlessness, swollen ankles) and heart conditions (IHD, MI, valvular heart disease, rheumatic fever).
  • Pulse rate and rhythm.
  • Circulatory status. Is the patient shut down? (low BP, cold peripheries, sweaty).
  • Signs of cardiac failure (raised JVP, peripheral oedema, basal inspiratory crackles, gallop rhythm—third and/or fourth heart sounds).
3 Do an ECG, and compare with previous ones.
4 Scan the patient's notes for details of current condition and treatment.

5 Document your findings and notify your senior.

Management of specific arrhythmias

Management of specific arrhythmias requires treatment of any underlying cause of cardiac decompensation, precise ECG diagnosis and correction of metabolic derangement. Use this section as a guide only. Local drug and consultant preference may markedly alter management. House Officers are not expected to diagnose or treat specific arrhythmias without senior advice.

Arrhythmias when the pulse is irregular with a NORMAL rate

Atrial fibrillation (normal rate)
Wandering atrial pacemaker
Ventricular ectopics
Variable AV block

On the ward

1 Severe symptoms are unusual. First do an ECG and then examine the patient. Atrial fibrillation and ectopics are common. Check the notes and find the most recent ECG for comparison. Is this a new problem?
2 In most cases, the arrhythmia is not significant. However, if the ECG reveals atrial fibrillation or multiple, frequent ectopics:
   • Examine the patient for heart failure (raised JVP, basal crackles, swollen ankles) and mitral valve disease (murmurs, added sounds, mitral facies).
   • Consider thyroid disease.
3 Investigations to consider:
   • C&E, FBC, ESR, serial cardiac enzymes.

• Serial ECGs (AF is common post-MI).
• Consider T$_4$, TSH, digoxin levels and an ECHO.
Discuss further management with your senior.

Hints

• A normal peripheral pulse may coexist with a fast central heart rate. Measure and document both.
• AF is associated with MI, IHD, mitral valve disease, thyroid disease, hypertension, pericarditis and other causes of a dilated atrium. Rarely, it is associated with atrial myxoma, infiltration, endocarditis and rheumatic fever. It is common following cardiac surgery, when it is usually temporary.

Arrhythmias when the pulse is irregular with a SLOW rate

Sinus bradycardia
Sudden stress, severe pain, post-systemic infection
Inferior MI
AV heart block
   Second degree heart block: intermittent block with or without an elongated P–R interval
   Third degree heart block: complete heart block (no relationship between P-waves and the QRS complex)
Drugs: amiodarone, beta-blockers, calcium channel blockers, digoxin
Faulty sinus node: sick sinus syndrome, infiltration
Hypothyroidism and hypothermia
Raised ICP
Jaundice

On the ward

1 See the patient and assess ABC. Bradycardic arrhythmias can be serious. *If flat*, call the crash team and start CPR if necessary. Give 100% O_2.

2 If the patient is stable but symptomatic, inform your senior and:
- Consider urgent ECG and C&E.
- Review all 'suspect' drugs (see above).
- If symptomatic with sinus bradycardia or AV block, give atropine 0.6 mg IV (up to 3 mg in 24 hours). If bradycardia continues, get help. Consider starting an isoprenaline infusion 1–3 µg/minute as a bridging measure while the patient waits for pacing.
- Consider urgent digoxin levels.

3 If the patient is asymptomatic, do an ECG and discuss further management with your senior.

Hints

- A fourth heart sound with bradycardia is common following inferior MI.
- A history of recent collapse requires urgent assessment even if the patient is currently asymptomatic.

Arrhythmias when the pulse is irregular with a FAST rate

Sinus tachycardia
- Hypermetabolic states, e.g. fever, anxiety, hyperthyroidism
- Drugs: digoxin, nitrates, nicotine, sympathomimetics, theophylline
- Shock, sepsis or hypovolaemia of any cause
- Heart failure

Supra-ventricular tachycardia
- Atrial flutter and fibrillation
- Paroxysmal atrial tachycardia
- WPW syndrome
- Nodal (junctional)
Ventricular tachycardia

On the ward

1 See the patient. Fast rate arrhythmias can be serious. Assess ABC. If flat, call the crash team, request an urgent ECG and start CPR if necessary. Give 100% O_2.

2 If the patient is stable, do an urgent ECG and consider a cardiac monitor. On the basis of the ECG, decide whether the patient has sinus tachycardia (normal wave form) or an arrhythmia.
- If the ECG reveals a sinus tachycardia, treat the underlying condition.
- If the ECG reveals an arrhythmia, you need to differentiate between SVT and VT, which can be difficult (see p. 41). Seek senior advice if you are unsure.

SVTs
- If the patient has SVT *and* hypotension, get help fast. The patient may require 50–100 J of DC conversion. Discuss transfer to CCU.
- The commonest cause of SVT without hypotension is atrial fibrillation (AF) (irregularly irregular pulse and no P waves on ECG). Common causes of fast AF in the hospital setting include MI, pulmonary embolus and pneumonia. First line treatment is digoxin or cardioversion if the AF is of acute onset. Digoxin controls the ventricular rate,

but does not cure the underlying fibrillation (see Drugs p. 101 for initiating digoxin therapy).

• If the patient has SVT that is not AF, they may need immediate treatment, but discuss with your senior first. Most SVTs respond to IV adenosine. Ensure that the patient is on a cardiac monitor and that a resus trolley is close to hand. Inject 3 mg adenosine rapidly into a large peripheral or central vein. If there is no response after 1–2 minutes, give 6 mg, and then a further 12 mg if necessary. Expect facial flushing, transient breathlessness and nausea.

VTs

• Sustained VT usually precipitates shock unless treated with DC conversion (100–200 J), so seek urgent senior help. Note that a broad complex tachycardia may be SVT with bundle branch block but should be treated as VT until proved otherwise.

• Investigations to consider:
    C&E, Ca, Mg, cardiac enzymes if recent onset, FBC if acutely unwell. Consider T_4 and TSH.
    Drug levels as appropriate: digoxin, theophylline and anti-arrhythmics. ABGs and CXR if acutely unwell.

Whether the patient has a VT or SVT, you need to identify and treat the underlying cause, in addition to treating the arrhythmia.

Hints

• In discriminating between SVT and VT:
    SVTs have narrow complexes (<140 ms) and are not necessarily associated with serious underlying heart disease.
    VTs have broad complexes (>140 ms)

and always indicates serious underlying heart disease.

• Carotid sinus massage can cause sinus arrest, especially in the elderly, or if the patient has had a recent MI or is digitalized. Use only if urgent action is required.

• Atrial tachycardia with heart block is commonly associated with digoxin toxicity.

Calcium

Most labs report *total* serum Ca, of which about half is bound to albumin. If the albumin levels are low the lab result will under-estimate total Ca. To correct roughly for hypoalbuminaemia, add *0.02 × the albumin deficit* to the laboratory result, or ask for an ionized Ca level which need not be adjusted for albumin (a special tube is required). Albumin deficit is defined as *40 − measured albumin level.*

Hypercalcaemia

On the wards, this is often spurious and often an incidental finding. However, true hypercalcaemia may need to be corrected. Rarely, it requires urgent treatment.

Differential diagnoses
• Spurious: tourniquet left on too long or blood taken from the drip arm
• Hyperparathyroidism (primary and tertiary)
• Malignancy – bony metastases, myeloma, paraneoplastic syndrome

continued on p. 42

• Drugs – thiazide diuretics, excessive ingestion of Ca-containing antacids, excessive vitamin D intake
• Rarer causes: granulomatous diseases (e.g. sarcoid, TB), endocrinopathies

On the ward

1 See the patient. Check that the result reflects true hypercalcaemia. In hospital, hypercalcaemia is usually an incidental finding and is frequently 'spurious', due to dehydration, venous stasis, taking blood from an infusion arm or abnormal albumin (see above). However, a corrected Ca of above 3.5 mmol/l usually requires treatment.
2 Exclude acute symptoms which require urgent treatment (anorexia, vomiting, abdominal pain, impaired mental state, dehydration). If acutely symptomatic:
    • Seek senior advice.
    • Consider: saline diuresis: 3–6 l normal saline/24 hours IV and frusemide 40–120 mg 2–4-hourly according to response. A CVP is useful to monitor fluid balance.
    • Avoid phosphates until Ca levels are normal or risk deposition of Ca phosphate ('metastatic Ca/Pi deposition').
    • Consider hydrocortisone (especially useful in malignancy, sarcoid and vitamin D intoxication), calcitonin or mithramycin therapy.
3 If the patient has true hypercalcaemia but is not acutely unwell:
    • If dehydrated, request that the patient drink enough fluid to maintain a urine output of >2–3 litres/day.

If very dehydrated or unable to drink, consider IV fluids.
• Investigate the cause of hypercalcaemia, exclude renal impairment and correct abnormal K and Mg levels (see investigations below).
• Mobilize as soon as possible.
4 Investigations to consider:
    • C&E, ESR, phosphate, alk phos, Mg.
    • ECG. Review CXR.
    • Consider plasma Igs, serum and urine electrophoresis, urinary Bence-Jones protein, skeletal survey, bone marrow biopsy (myeloma investigations) and PTH levels.

Hypocalcaemia

Like hypercalcaemia, hypocalcaemia can be spurious and may be caused by acute hyperventilation. Hypocalcaemia is rarely an emergency, unless Ca is <1.5 mmol/l (risking laryngospasm).

Differential diagnoses
• Spurious (low albumin, blood taken from drip arm)
• Acute hyperventilation
• Major systemic illness, especially pancreatitis
• Hypoparathyroidism – thyroid surgery or neck irradiation
• On TPN without adequate Ca
• Vitamin D deficiency – malabsorption, renal disease, phenytoin or phenobarbitone
• Excessive ingestion of phosphate

On the ward

1 Assess the severity of the patient's

condition. Check that the result is not spurious. Look for peripheral or oral paraesthesia, carpo-pedal spasm, Chvostek's sign (tapping over the facial nerve induces facial twitch), confusion and tetany.

2 If hypocalcaemia is symptomatic or Ca <1.5 mmol/l, seek immediate senior advice and institute treatment to prevent laryngo-spasm. Give 10% Ca gluconate 10–20 ml in 50–100 ml 5% dextrose over 5 minutes (not faster), followed by 1–2 mg/kg/h IV for 6–12 hours according to response. Correct the Mg deficiency and measure the phosphate level. If the phosphate is high, discuss with senior. The patient may need phosphate binders and slow correction of Ca, as too rapid correction can result in metastatic deposition of Ca phosphate.

3 Asymptomatic hypocalcaemia (Ca >1.75 mmol/l) does not require immediate treatment. Give oral supplements (2–4 g daily in divided doses) that contain cholecalciferol (most do – see the *BNF*).

4 Investigations to consider:
  • C&E, Mg, phosphate.
  • Others according to the differential diagnosis.

Hint

• To avoid hypocalcaemia in patients on TPN, check Mg and Ca measurements at least weekly, and more frequently if acutely unwell.

Chest pain

Chest pain always requires urgent atten-tion. While angina, oesophagitis and oesophageal spasm are the commonest causes of chest pain, never forget pulmonary embolus in the hospital setting.

When answering your bleep

Ask the ward staff to:
• Find an ECG machine.
• Repeat the vital signs.
• If the patient has a history of IHD, prescribe sub-lingual GTN 5 mg over the phone and start 40% O_2.

Differential diagnoses
Heart
• Angina (IHD, LVH/HOCM)
• Acute MI
• Pericarditis, including post-MI Dressler's syndrome

Lung/pleura
• Pulmonary embolus
• Pneumothorax
• Pleurisy/pneumonia

Aorta
• Dissection
• Aneurysm

GIT
• Oesophageal spasm
• Oesophagitis/gastritis
• Pancreatitis, cholecystitis, peptic ulcer

Other
• Shingles
• Costochondritis
• Rib or vertebral collapse

continued on p. 44

Sudden onset of central chest pain
• Exacerbation of IHD
• MI
• Oesophageal spasm
• PE or dissecting aneurysm
• Pneumothorax

On the ward

1 Assess the patient. If flat, get help (+/− crash team) and institute emergency treatment:
   • 100% O_2.
   • IV access.
   • Urgent C&E, FBC, cardiac enzymes, ABGs.
   • ECG (stat) and ECG monitor.
   • Urgent mobile CXR.
2 If the patient is stable, take a more thorough history and examination. Don't forget:
   • T, BP, pulse and circulation (well-perfused or cold and clammy?).
   • The key to the diagnosis is the history. Specifically:
   (a) Ask a lot about the pain itself. Have they had this pain before? Do they have known IHD or oesophagitis/oesophageal spasm? Does the pain feel anginal? Is it relieved by GTN? Relieving or precipitating factors (exercise, posture, food)? Pain lasting less than 30 seconds, stabbing or sharp in quality and highly localized is unlikely to be due to ischaemia.
   (b) Any N&V (common with MI)? Recent falls or trauma?
   • Listen for pleural and pericardial rubs (often missed).
   • If there are odd chest noises, think of pneumothorax.
3 Investigations to consider:
   • ECG +/− CXR.
   • IV access if you suspect an MI.

• Repeat ECG in 1–2 hours (there may be no ECG changes in an early MI).
• C&E and cardiac enzymes. Consider blood gases, FBC, clotting and G&S if embolus, anticoagulation or surgery is likely.
4 Discuss with your senior.

Hints

• Pain radiating to either arm, neck or jaw suggests a cardiac cause.
• Sub-lingual GTN provides immediate relief of angina and is a useful diagnostic aid. It also relieves oesophageal spasm, but over a few minutes.
• Oesophageal spasm or severe anxiety sometimes causes ischaemic-like changes on the ECG. Seek advice if unsure.

Confusion

Beware of unexpected confusion in patients. In particular, hypoxia is common but easily missed in the elderly. Never assume disorientation or dementia without first excluding serious medical causes and ascertaining the patient's usual mental state.

When answering your bleep ask for

• A ward blood glucose test (blood glucose stick).
• T, BP, pulse and urine dipstick.
• Pulse oximetry if available (p. 74).

Differential diagnoses
'DIM TOP' (Mike's South African acronym!)

continued

Drugs (especially sedatives and analgesics)

Infection (anywhere; commonly UTI and pneumonia)

Metabolic – hypoglycaemia, Na+, K+, Ca, liver or renal failure

Trauma (concussion, subdural haematoma)

Toxins (alcohol withdrawal, drugs, others)

Oxygen deficit (hypoxia) – pneumonia, PE, respiratory depression (opiates), anaemia

Pain and discomfort (any cause, including urinary/faecal retention)

Psychiatric/dementia

Perfusion abnormalities (CVA, TIA)

Post-op confusion (hypoxia, urinary retention, infection, drugs, abnormal electrolytes, pain, blood loss, disorientation, alcohol withdrawal)

On the ward

1 Assess the patient's general condition and vital signs. If the patient is very agitated or violent, get help from nurses and porters. Consider sedation (5 mg diazepam IV is usually sufficient). Alternatively, use 5–10 mg haloperidol IM or PO or chlorpromazine 50–100 mg IM or PO (caution in cardiac patients). Have a resus trolley to hand. You may need to wait 10–20 minutes for the drug to take effect. In alcoholic patients consider chlormethiazole instead (see p. 104).

2 If the patient is stable, take a history and examination. Don't forget to:

- Specifically exclude cardiac and respiratory distress. Breathe with the patient and consider a pulse oximeter reading or ABGs. Hypoxia is a surprisingly common cause of confusion that is easily missed.
- Perform a mini-mental test score. Is the patient truly confused or just disorientated, in pain or angry?
- Ask about recent falls, funny turns or previous strokes/TIAs. Is the patient in atrial fibrillation?
- Check possible infection sites (IV lines, UTI, chest, surgical wounds) and palpate for a full bladder or packed colon (urinary retention is a common cause of confusion). Look at the fundi for raised ICP (e.g. in subdural haematoma) and briefly assess the CNS for localizing signs.
- Check drug and fluid charts and review the medical background.

3 Ask the nursing staff or a relative about the patient's usual mental state. Is this a new occurrence?

4 Investigations to consider:
- C&E, Glucose, FBC and ESR,
- ABGs,
- Blood cultures,
- Liver function tests (INR),
- Plasma Ca in patients with malignancy.
- MSU.
- ECG.
- CXR, CT head.

Hints

- Nurse the patient in a moderately lit room and minimize noise. Give repeated reassurance to the patient. A well-loved family member or a familiar nurse is invaluable.
- Consider nursing the patient on a mattress on the floor. Some hospitals have special 'soft walled' beds. Bed rails

and 'hand ties' are regarded by most nursing staff as unnecessary and potentially dangerous.

• Secure NG tubes and IV lines with bandages. It is occasionally necessary to put mittens on the patient's hands.

• If you have excluded serious causes, consider short-term sedation with a benzodiazepine (diazepam 5–10 mg IV slowly, repeated 4-hourly if necessary). For shorter effect use lorazepam 1–2 mg (25–30 µg/kg) IV slowly, repeated after 6 hours if necessary. Use with caution in the elderly. Alternatives include:

Haloperidol 5–10 mg IM or PO

Chlorpromazine 50–100 mg IM or PO (caution in cardiac patients). (Both haloperidol and chlorpromazine are especially useful in the more acute setting. Have a resus trolley to hand. You may need to wait 10–20 minutes for the drug to take effect).

In alcoholic patients consider chlormethiazole instead (see p. 104).

Thioridazine 12.5–25 mg PO at night or 12 hourly is often used in geriatric units.

• You may not find any cause for the patient's confusion. Patients may simply be disorientated from a change in environment, but make sure you exclude serious medical causes before making this diagnosis. Clear, repeated explanation about where the patient is and why can be helpful, as is a small map showing where the toilets are and how to call for nursing assistance.

Constipation

Constipation is very common in hospital due to hospital food, immobility, drugs and having to use a bedpan. It is more effective to treat the cause than to prescribe laxatives. Always be alert to obstruction and its causes (particularly tumours). Post-op ileus is common, usually resolves by itself and should never be treated with laxatives!

Differential diagnoses

Low roughage diet

Immobility

Drugs

• Aluminium or Ca-based drugs (e.g. antacids)

• Ca channel blockers (verapamil)

• Ferrous sulphate

• Opiates

• Tricyclic antidepressants

• Anticholinergics

• Slow K+

Embarrassment at using a bedpan

GIT

• Pain (anal fissures, haemorrhoids, recent surgery)

• IBS

• Obstruction (acute and sub-acute) from any cause, especially tumours

• Ileus (pseudo-obstruction)

Metabolic

• Dehydration (especially in the elderly)

• Endocrine – hypothyroidism

• Hypercalcaemia, hypokalaemia

Neurological

• Spinal cord compression/lesions

On the ward

1 See the patient. Exclude:

• Intestinal obstruction (vomiting, abdominal pain or distension, high pitched bowel sounds). If present, consider tumour (see p. 36 Abdominal pain).

• IBD (which can cause constipation. Never prescribe laxatives in these patients without first consulting your senior).

• Pain or embarrassment which may inhibit straining. Have they had recent surgery?

2 Take a brief history and examination. Don't forget:

• To ask the patient how often they usually open their bowels. They may not have true constipation.

• PR (faecal impaction, anal fissure). Check for FOB.

• Drug and fluid charts.

3 Investigations are seldom necessary but consider:

• K+, Ca, FBC.

• T_4 and TSH only if you suspect hypothyroidism.

4 Management. For simple constipation:

• Ensure adequate hydration and mobilize if possible.

• Bulk-forming agents: bran cereals or ispaghula husk (Fybogel or Metamucil).

• Stool softeners: ducosate sodium (cheap) or lactulose (expensive).

• Stimulants: senna or bisacodyl. Glycerine suppositories if NBM. Codanthrusate (danthron docusate) is very effective but reserved for very elderly or terminally ill patients due to risk of danthron induced GIT tumours.

• Enemas, e.g. phosphate enema 100 ml.

5 Consider prophylaxis for patients at risk of constipation (bedridden, e.g. post-op, CVA or patients on regular opiates):

• Stool softeners (docusate sodium 100 mg/day, or lactulose 10 ml/bd) and/or stimulants (senna 1–2 tablets daily) or enemas. Adjust doses in light of symptoms.

Diarrhoea

By far the commonest cause in hospital is drugs (antibiotics and laxatives) but infection should always be considered. Less common but important to consider is obstruction with overflow. In all cases, the patient may need to be rehydrated.

Differential diagnoses

• Anxiety and pain

• Drugs: laxatives, broad-spectrum antibiotics leading to *Clostridium difficile* infection (pseudo-membranous colitis), antacids containing Mg sulphate. Also cimetidine, colchicine, cytotoxic agents, digoxin, thiazide diuretics (see the *BNF*)

   intestinal obstruction with overflow (neoplasm)

• Faecal impaction with overflow, especially in elderly patients

• Infection (immunocompromised? antibiotics? recent travel?)

• IBD, other causes of intra-abdominal inflammation, ischaemia, etc.

• Non-specific in association with other diseases

On the ward

1 Exclude severe dehydration (vital signs: BP lying and sitting, JVP, mucous membranes).

2 Directed history and examination:

• Risk for intra-abdominal sepsis (recent surgery, diverticular disease), IBD, immunocompromise (including HIV).

- N&V, blood or mucus PR.
- Peritonism or impaction.
- Drug chart for new drugs, laxatives, antibiotics.

3 If the patient is otherwise well, and an infective cause is unlikely with no evidence of colitis or intra-abdominal mischief, send a stool sample for MC&S and prescribe an antidiarrhoeal agent, e.g. loperamide 4 mg initially, then 2 mg with each loose stool.

4 If the patient has systemic signs or is taking antibiotics:
- Take a fresh stool specimen (¥3) for MC&S and *Clostridium difficile* toxin.
- Consider sigmoidoscopy and biopsy if the patient has bloody diarrhoea or the stool culture is negative.

5 Further investigations to consider:
- C&E; FBC to check WCC
  Electron microscopy (EM) of stool specimen for viral infection (SSRVs)
  Inflammatory markers (CRP and ESR) especially if known IBD.
  Special cultures/stains for cryptosporidia, mycobacteria, etc. for immunocompromised patients.

6 Irrespective of the cause you must ensure adequate hydration.
- Oral rehydration regime (see *BNF*—oral rehydration).
- IV fluids if severe or the patient cannot drink (see p. 58).

Hints

- Barrier nursing is advisable until infection is ruled out.
- Always wash your hands between patients.
- Be wary of diarrhoea in patients on steroids. Their abdomens may be 'silent' despite serious intra-abdominal mischief.

Electrocardiograms

Don't get too worried about interpreting ECGs during your house job. While the range of potential anomalies is bewildering at first, practice really does make perfect and House Officers are only expected to diagnose a handful of important conditions (see below). For a more complete guide consult Hampton's *ECG Made Easy* and *ECG in Practice* (see Bibliography, p. 2). Whatever the ECG diagnosis, remember to treat the patient, not the ECG!

Common ECG diagnoses

Atrial fibrillation (no P waves, rate can be fast or normal)
Recent or past MI (see below)
Third degree heart block (no relationship between P waves and QRS complexes)
Ventricular tachycardia
Ventricular fibrillation

Basic ECG parameters to consider

- Rate: 60–90 bpm (lower in athletes)
- Rhythm: irregular or regular
- Axis: normal: −30 to +120° (some use 0 to +90)
- P waves: present/absent before each QRS complex?
- PR interval: constant? Normal 120–200 ms (3–5

continued

	small squares)
• QRS complexes:	up to 120 ms (3 small squares). Check height of the R waves
	Are Q waves present?
• ST segment:	isoelectric (i.e. on baseline)?
• T waves:	upright or inverted?

If the ECG is abnormal, consider each parameter systematically:

Abnormal rate and rhythm

Atrial tachycardia

• QRS rate >100/minute.
• Perhaps narrow QRS (<120 ms) (except in SVT with BBB or WPW syndrome).
• P wave abnormal (shape, size, upside down, swallowed by QRS, or with short PR interval).

Atrial fibrillation

• No P waves.
• Irregularly timed QRS complexes.

Atrial flutter

• Saw-tooth baseline of atrial depolarization.
• Regular QRS complexes.

AV nodal rhythm

• Narrow QRS complex.
• P waves hidden within the QRS complex or just preceding it (very short PR interval).

Ventricular tachycardia

• Wide QRS (>120 ms), rate >150/minute.
• Abnormal T waves.
• P waves often absent or may have no relationship to QRS complexes.

Hint

• If there is a rapid QRS rate without P waves, a wide QRS (>120 ms) indicates VT (unless there is pre-existing BBB) whereas a narrow QRS (<120 ms) indicates AV nodal tachycardia.

Calculating the axis

1 If the QRS is predominantly positive in I and II the axis is normal.
2 If not, find a lead in which the QRS complexes have equal positive and negative deflections. The axis lies 90° to that lead.
3 To determine the actual axis see Fig. 7.1.

P waves

1 Indicate atrial depolarization and are best seen in leads II and V1.
2 Large left atrium (p. mitrale): bifid and wide (>110 ms), P wave in II, biphasic in V1.
3 Large right atrium (p. pulmonale): peaked P waves (>2.5 mm). Look at lead II.
4 No P waves: atrial fibrillation.

PR interval

Delay indicates abnormal AV conduction = HB.

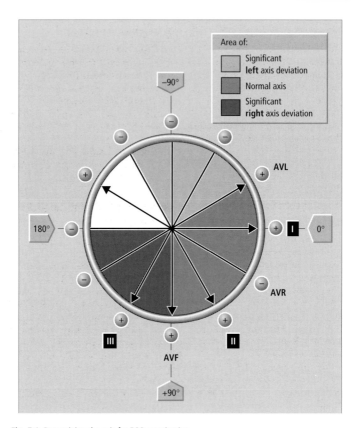

Fig. 7.1 Determining the axis for ECG examination.

1 First degree HB: prolonged PR interval in each cycle but all P waves conducted.
2 Second degree HB: some P waves are not followed by a QRS complex. May find 2 (or 3) P waves before a QRS complex = 2:1 (or 3:1) block. P wave rate is normal. Progressive lengthening of the PR interval then non-conducted P wave is called the Wenckebach phenomenon.
3 Third degree HB: no relationship between P waves and QRS complexes. Ventricular escape rhythm <50/minute. QRS usually wide.
4 A consistently short PR interval indicates conduction down accessory pathways (e.g. WPW).

QRS complexes

Wide complexes (>120 ms) indicate abnormal ventricular depolarization, occurring in VT, ventricular extra-systoles, complete heart block or bundle branch block.

1 Ventricular extra-systoles: no P-wave, early QRS and abnormally shaped QRS complex, abnormal T-wave. Next P wave is 'on time'.

2 LBBB: RSR' 'W' pattern in V1, 'M' pattern in V6. Inverted T waves in I, a VL, V5–6. The presence of LBBB may mask underlying infarction.

3 RBBB: RSR' 'M' pattern in V1, 'W' pattern in V6. Inverted T waves in V1–3, deep and wide S wave in V6.

4 Ventricular strain/hypertrophy: inverted T waves and depressed ST segments in the appropriate chest leads (V1–3 for RV and V4–6 for LV).

5 RVH: R wave larger than S wave in V1 and no RBBB, deep S in V6. Sometimes right axis deviation. NB: a dominant R in V1 is seen in posterior infarction and RBBB.

6 LVH: R wave in V6 >25 mm in height; R wave in V6 + S wave in V1 >35 mm in height. Occasionally left axis deviation.

ST segment and T waves

1 Depressed ST segments: ischaemia, digoxin toxicity ('inverted tick' ST depression and inverted T waves in V5–6).

2 Elevated ST segments (always serious): infarction, coronary artery spasm (variant angina), pericarditis (saddle-shaped ST segments in all leads), ventricular aneurysm.

3 T wave inversion is often non-specific but in the context of chest pain points to critical ischaemia.

Important ECG abnormalities to recognize

Myocardial infarction. Sequence of changes (Table 7.2):

1 At first the ECG may be normal.

2 Within 6 hours, tall T waves and raised ST segments are evident.

3 Within 24 hours, T waves invert and ST segments normalize.

4 After 24 hours, Q waves are evident and ST segments are normal.

NB: T wave inversion may or may not persist. Q waves persist.

Pulmonary embolism. There are often no ECG changes:

Table 7.2 Diagnosing infarction sites by ECG changes.

Site of infarction	Changes seen in leads
Anterior	V2–V5
Inferior	III and a VF
Lateral	I, a VL and V6
True posterior	Dominant R in V1 (exclude RV strain and RBBB)

1 Sinus tachycardia.
2 Evidence of RV strain/hypertrophy (see above).
3 Right axis deviation.
4 RBBB.
5 Deep S in I, Q in V3, inverted T in V3 ('SI, Q3, T3').

Eye complaints

Except for the simplest problems, House Officers are not expected to diagnose or treat eye diseases. Do not be afraid to seek an ophthalmological opinion. Ophthalmologists are usually keen for referrals and can teach you a lot.

The acute red eye

Differential diagnoses
Conjunctivitis
Foreign body
Corneal ulceration/herpes keratitis
Acute glaucoma
Acute iritis

On the ward

1 Take a brief history and examination. Don't forget:
  • Clinical background, especially diabetes and other systemic diseases.
  • Visual acuity, discharge, corneal lustre.
  • Pupils: shape, direct and consensual responses.
  • Ophthalmoscopy to assess red reflex (normal in conjuctivitis and simple foreign body) and fundus.
2 Unless the cause is obvious, notify your senior and seek an urgent ophthalmological opinion.
  • If the problem is unilateral, ask about previous history of shingles (look for periocular vesicles) or iritis (which often recurs in the fellow eye). Conjunctivitis or ulceration can also be unilateral.
• Exclude conjunctivitis: the eye usually feels itchy and tears. Vision, corneal lustre, pupillary responses and red-reflex are all normal. Purulent discharge suggests bacterial conjunctivitis. Look at the pattern of redness/injection. Intensity of injection around the periphery suggests conjunctival inflammation, whereas injection around the cornea suggests corneal or intra-ocular inflammation.
• Exclude acute glaucoma: the eye is red and painful, the pupil is hazy and fixed and the patient sees halos around lights. Seek urgent ophthalmological assistance.
• Exclude a foreign body: the eye usually tears. Foreign bodies are sometimes hidden under the inside of the upper lid. Invert the upper lid over a small spatula (cotton bud or orange stick). Bear in mind that the sensation of having a foreign body in the eye can also be caused by corneal ulcers and acute keratitis.

Sudden loss of vision

This is always an emergency. Seek immediate ophthalmological advice.

Differential diagnoses
Acute glaucoma
Central artery or vein occlusion
Optic neuritis
Retinal detachment
Severe hyperglycaemia
Temporal arteritis

Floaters

Floaters are usually condensations of vitreous, but can be blood, bits of retina or inflammatory cells. They are normal with age, but if they have appeared recently or suddenly, seek an ophthalmological opinion.

Falls

While most falls in hospital are trivial, they are a common cause of fracture in the elderly. You need to sign an accident form when called to investigate a 'fall' (see p. 10).

When answering your bleep

• Consider asking for a ward glc test.

Differential diagnoses

• Simple accident (slippery floor, disorientation, frailty, generalized weakness from illness)
• Poor vision (no glasses, cataracts)
• Drowsiness from drugs, especially sedatives and recent anaesthesia

Occasionally:

• Loss of consciousness: TIA, fit, vaso-vagal, postural hypotension, vasodilator and other drugs, cough/micturition syncope, arrhythmias/MI, PE, mitral/aortic stenosis, hypoglycaemia, anaemia
• Poor motor function/balance: generalized weakness from illness, Parkinson's disease, cerebellar disease, peripheral neuropathy, myasthenia gravis

On the ward

1 See the patient. Nurses are legally liable until the patient is seen by a doctor.
2 Ask the patient what happened and which part hurts the most. Don't forget:
   • T, pulse and BP, including postural drop.
   • Consciousness level (see Glasgow Coma Scale, p. 208) and mini-mental test score if appropriate.
   • Skin for bruising, bleeding, cuts and fractures.
   • Bone tenderness for fractures. Frail patients can sustain fractures with remarkably little fuss. Especially look for hip, wrist and scaphoid fractures. Examine the skull carefully if the patient has hit their head. If there are signs of head injury or drowsiness, consider a CT head (see p. 176).
   • Drug and fluid charts (sedatives, hypoglycaemic agents, vasodilators (especially ACE inhibitors), antiarrhythmics).
3 Investigations to consider:
   • C&E, FBC (?raised WCC), glucose.
   • MSU.
   • ECG.
   • The patient may need cardiac investigations later (e.g. ECHO, 24-hour ECG).
4 Sign an accident form (ask the nurses for one). If the patient appears well, 'No apparent injuries on examination' is sufficient.
5 Write in the patient's notes. Include:
   • Time and date.
   • Brief history of accident.
   • Brief examination findings.

• That you signed an accident form.

6 Ask the nurses to continue to do regular observations and to contact you if the patient's condition deteriorates. If the patient has hit their head, consider requesting neurological observations.

7 Think about what caused the fall. Make a plan with the nurses to prevent future accidents.

Hints

• Many falls are caused by patients being in an alien environment, particularly in elderly patients with poor righting reflexes. To prevent future falls, show patients the call button and remind them that they need to call the nurse for toilet assistance after anaesthetics or sedatives. If the bed needs to remain raised high off the floor, caution patients about the drop before stepping down onto slippery linoleum.

• Fractures or simple bruising in the elderly can lead to substantial blood loss, Never forget to check limbs for occult fractures.

• Sudden loss of consciousness is most commonly caused by fainting, postural hypotension and arrhythmia. MIs rarely present with syncope alone.

Fever

In hospital, fever is most commonly due to infection, blood transfusions and drugs. When called at night, the major concern is to exclude bacterial infection.

Differential diagnosis

Infection, especially UTI, phlebitis, pneumonia. More common in diabetics

Drug-induced, especially antibiotics, allopurinol, ibuprofen. Common during blood transfusions

Thrombosis +/− infarction: DVT, PE, MI, ischaemic bowel

Tumours

Alcohol withdrawal

Hyperthyroidism

Inflammatory and vasculitides, especially IBD, rheumatoid arthritis

Post-surgery

Think 4 Ws: Wind, Wound (including lines), Water, Walking (DVT).

On the ward

1 See the patient. Check T, pulse and BP and check the charts. Fever above 40 °C requires urgent action. If there is any chance of shock (tachycardia, hypotension with warm peripheries), ensure large-bore IV access and commence IV fluid resuscitation. Take blood cultures (at least two sets). Discuss IV broad-spectrum antibiotic cover with your senior.

2 Exclude immunosuppression and diabetes. Check the patient's history, latest WCC and glucose. In either case, look vigorously for infection site (see p. 56).

3 Try to localize the source of infection. Don't forget to consider:

• Asking about abdominal pain, cough, chest pain, diarrhoea, dysuria/frequency, prosthesis/heart valves, rashes, rigors/chills.

Table 7.3 Common postoperative causes of fever.

Day 1–2	Day 2–4	Day 5–10
Atelectasis +/- infection	DVT	As for days 1–4
Aspiration pneumonia	PE	Deep abscess formation
UTI	Wound infections	

• Recent surgery or invasive procedure?

• Recent sexual contacts, travel abroad (TB, malaria, amoebiasis)?

• Drugs

Common sites for infection:

• Chest, wound/line sites, bladder.

• Skin, leg ulcers.

• ENT (remember ears). Check for meningism.

• IV lines, catheters, drains – how long have these been in place?

• Do not forget to examine the genitalia, do a PR (ischiorectal/prostatic abscess), and consider PV (PID). Check joints for tenderness and swelling.

4 Consider other diagnostic possibilities (see Table 7.3). Check the legs, as DVTs are easily missed.

5 Investigations to consider:

• Urine dipstick and MSU.

• FBC +/− white cell differential. C&E, CRP, ESR. Blood gases or pulse oximetry if you suspect a PE or pneumonia.

• Blood cultures.

Consider further investigations:

• Other cultures (sputum, stool, CSF, wound swabs, catheter tips).

• Radiology (CXR, AXR, sinus X-ray, US, CT scan, ECHO).

• Serology.

6 Management. Take cultures and decide whether or not to start antibiotics straight away:

• You should start antibiotics if the patient is immunocompromised or diabetic as these patients can deteriorate rapidly. See p. 56.

• If the patient is otherwise well, has a T of <38.5 °C and is not immunocompromised or diabetic, you can usually prescribe an antipyretic and withhold antibiotics until you have test results (e.g. WCC). Have the nurses call you if the T rises and discuss with your senior if in doubt. Conservative management is usually appropriate for patients in the following circumstances, if their T is <38.5 °C:

• Up to 24 hours post-op or following invasive procedures.

• Following blood transfusion (see p. 81).

• If antibiotics started in the past 24 hours.

• Paracetamol (1 g 4–6-hourly) is a good antipyretic. For fevers above 40 °C, prescribe tepid sponging and fanning.

• If SBE is a possibility you need to take three sets of blood cultures from different sites and at different times (3–6 hours apart). Do not start antibiotics before consulting with your senior, as starting antibiotics before a diagnosis is confirmed may prevent isolation of an organism which makes effective treatment much more difficult.

• Remember to make best use of your microbiology department. They are usually eager to help you.

The immunocompromised patient with fever

A patients is defined as immunocompromised if they: have WCC $<2 \times 10^9/l$, an absolute neutrophil count $< 1 \times 10^9/l$ (neutropenia), are HIV-positive with a low CD4 count, are on high dose steroids or other immunosuppressants.

On the ward

1 Take a quick history and examination (see above) remembering:
    • The patient can have weird organisms in weird places, including CNS.
    • Check *all* orifices.
    • They can deteriorate rapidly (within hours). Seek senior advice early.
2 Investigations:
    • Culture everything!
    • If there is a central line, take peripheral and central blood cultures (include a culture from each lumen of triple lumen cannulae).
    • Stool, urine, sputum, MSU and wound swabs, including from around the entry site of indwelling IV lines. Get advice from a microbiologist for special stains and cultures of sputum and stools for AFBs, PCP, *Cryptosporidium*, etc. if HIV-positive.

• Consider removing lines and culturing the tips (cut using sterile technique (sterile scissors, gloves) and send to microbiology in a sterile container). Discuss with senior.
• Re-check FBC for neutrophil count, platelets and Hb.
• C&E and glucose. Consider amylase, G&S, clotting, ESR, CRP.
• CXR (mobile).
• Specimen for serology if new patient.
3 Commence broad-spectrum antibiotics once cultures are taken. Antibiotic policy changes rapidly, so check the latest protocol with a microbiologist or pharmacist. An aminoglycoside plus piperacillin, with or without extra anaerobic cover (metronidazole), is usual. Add flucloxacillin if a staphylococcal wound or line infection is likely.

Fits

Your aim is to prevent the patient from harming themselves and to end the fit as soon as possible. Most fits last less than 5 minutes and do not require active treatment, but prolonged fits require urgent treatment to prevent hypoxia and brain damage.

When answering your bleep

• Ask for a ward glucose to be done.
• Note the time you were called and rush to the ward.

Differential diagnoses
Epilepsy and omitted anti-epileptic doses

continued

Drug or alcohol withdrawal
Hypoxia (fever in children)
CVA, sub-arachnoid haemorrhage
Infection or inflammation of the brain
    and meninges
Metabolic causes: hypoglycaemia
    or suprahyperglycaemia, deranged
    Ca, Mg, Na, thyroxine, urea,
    bilirubin (liver/renal failure)
Post-traumatic (sub-dural haema-
    toma)
Drug overdose—tricyclics, phe-
    nothiazines, amphetamines
About half are idiopathic

On the ward

1 Place the patient in the recovery position. Protect the patient's head with a
pillow.
2 Do not forcibly restrain the patient as
it tends to prolong the fit.
  • Give 100% O_2 by face-mask and
  insert an oral airway if possible, but
  never force one. The risk of choking
  on the tongue is less than that of
  choking on a tooth!
  • Establish IV access using a butterfly needle. Get help if you are struggling.
  • Give 5–10 mg diazepam (IV bolus)
  or rectal diazepam (10 mg) if IV
  access is impossible. If the fit does
  not terminate within 5 minutes of
  IV therapy, repeat diazepam 5 mg/
  minute up to 20 mg or until significant respiratory depression
  occurs.
  • If not already done, check blood
  glucose with blood glucose stick. If
  the patient is hypoglycaemic (glucose
  <2.5) give 50 ml of 50% glucose IV
  immediately. Flush the line with

saline. Alternatively give glucagon
(1–2 mg IM or SC).
3 If the patient is still fitting, call your
senior. Meanwhile, if the patient is not
already dosed with it, give phenytoin
1000–1500 mg (15–18 mg/kg) IV slowly
(not exceeding 50 mg/minute). Watch
for hypotension. If the patient has been
taking phenytoin, the next step is
phenobarbitone (15–20 mg/kg IV
slowly (up to 100 mg/minute) or IM) –
but get senior advice first. The patient
may need to be ventilated.
4 Once the fit has terminated:
  • Examine the patient for localizing
  CNS signs, evidence of raised ICP
  (check fundi, BP and pulse).
  • The patient will probably sleep
  deeply for some time.
  • Consider consequences for the patient's driving licence (see p. 212).
5 Investigations to consider:
  • FBC, C&E, blood glucose, liver
  biochemistry, Ca, Mg.
  • ABGs.
  • Blood cultures if febrile
  • CXR
  • LP if suspected bacterial
  meningitis
  • CT scan if the cause is unclear
  and there are localizing neurological signs, papilloedema or head
  injury.
  • Toxicology screen if indicated by
  the history
  • Blood for anticonvulsant levels
  (some hospitals can do these within
  an hour).

Hints

  • If you arrive after the patient has
  stopped fitting but it sounds like a typical grand mal seizure, discuss prophy-

laxis with your seniors. If known epileptic, consider why they fitted now:
  Does it fit with their usual pattern of seizures
  Intercurrent infection
  Alcohol abuse
  Poor compliance.
• A useful alternative to phenytoin (especially for alcoholics) is a ready-mixed 0.8% chlormethiazole solution for IV infusion; run in 40–100 ml over 5–10 minutes.
  If you suspect malnourishment or chronic alcohol abuse, give thiamine 100 mg IV.

Intravenous fluids

If you have never done it before, prescribing IV fluids can look horribly complicated. It isn't, providing you keep an eye out for the cardinal sins of IV hydration:
1 Over-hydration, risking heart failure.
2 Electrolyte imbalance, especially Na and K.
3 Phlebitis.
4 Unnecessary and expensive if the patient can drink!

How to prescribe IV fluids

1 Decide on the daily volume of fluid required:

• Look at the fluid chart each day to make sure that you are keeping up with (and not grossly exceeding) daily losses. Remember that in addition to recorded losses (urine, faeces, vomit), people lose 500 ml/24 hours in insensible losses.
• The average person needs 2–3 litres/24 hours (each litre given 8-hourly).
2 Decide on which fluid(s) to use:
Most patients can be given a daily total of 2–3 litres of fluid in ratio of 2 litres of 5% dextrose water to 1 litre of normal (0.9%) saline. These should contain a total of 40 mmol of K and 60–120 mmol Na in 24 hours. This is typically written up as shown in Table 7.4.
3 Exceptions:
• Replace saline with dextrose water in patients with liver failure or ascites.
• Avoid dextrose water in patients recovering from DKA or with hyponatraemia.
• K imbalance is easy to achieve with IV fluids – and easy to correct. Measure electrolytes daily and adjust the K accordingly. If the K is suddenly very high, repeat the sample. Spurious hyperkalaemia can occur if you take blood from the drip arm, leave the tourniquet on too long or haemolyse the cells.
• Hyponatraemia is a common and

Table 7.4 Example of typical fluid chart.

Date	Time	Fluid	Volume (ml)	Signature
1/1/96	8 hours	Normal saline + 20 mmol KCl	1000	J. Bloggs
1/1/96	8 hours	5% dextrose	1000	J. Bloggs
1/1/96	8 hours	5% dextrose + 20 mmol KCl	1000	J. Bloggs

Table 7.5 A rough guide to the electrolyte content and daily production of body fluids.

Fluid	Na⁺ (mmol)	Cl⁻ (mmol)	K⁺ (mmol)	HCO₃⁻ (mmol)	Daily (ml)
Sweat	50	40	5	–	Variable
Gastric	60–100	100	10	–	1500–2000
Bile	140	100	5	15–30	200–800
Pancreas	140	75	5	70–120	200–800
Ileum	140	100	5	15–30	2000–3000
Diarrhoea	50	40	35	45	Variable

potentially lethal complication of IV hydration. If the patent's Na begins to creep below 135 mmol/l, the first step is to reduce the total IV fluid load and substitute dextrose with normal saline (see Hyponatraemia p. 80).

Hints

• Patients with fever require about 10% more fluid for every degree Celsius above normal 37 °C.
• At least daily, examine elderly patients for signs of fluid overload and reduce fluids if necessary. Check the fluid charts and request daily weighing.
• See Table 7.5 for a rough guide to body fluid content.

Upper gastrointestinal bleeds

Always attend to GI bleed calls urgently as these patients can deteriorate rapidly, and apparently small bleeds can herald major bleeds. However, most reported bleeds are minor and do not require urgent action.

While answering your bleep

• Ask for BP and pulse to be taken as you head for the ward.

On the ward

The basic approach for all upper GI bleeds is the same:
1 See the patient. Assess the severity of the bleed. If the patient is hypovolaemic or at high risk for a major bleed (see box below), then they will require urgent treatment. To assess for severe hypovolaemia, check the BP, pulse and JVP (pulse >100/minute, sweaty and pale, cold peripheries, postural drop >20 mmHg and JVP imperceptible when lying at 30° or less).

High risk patients
Age >60 years
Haematemesis *and* melaena
Severe bleed
Re-bleed in same admission

continued

Patients on anticoagulant therapy
Co-existant cardiac, respiratory or
  renal failure
Known or suspected oesophageal
  varices or cirrhosis

High risk and hypovolaemic patients

If the patient is hypovolaemic or a high risk patient

1 Notify your senior immediately.
2 Remove false teeth. If hypotensive, give 100% O_2 and lower the patient's head.
3 Insert two cannulae (one in either arm), as big-bored as you can manage, even if the patient's bleeding seems to have stopped.
4 If the pulse is greater than 100 bpm or there are other signs of a major bleed, give 500 ml of colloid (Haemaccel) or 5% dextrose water as fast as possible and repeat if necessary while waiting for blood.
5 Urgently cross-match 4–6 units of blood. Use O-negative blood if the patient is still unstable after 3 units of colloid and a cross-match is not available.
6 Do FBC and clotting studies. Transfuse until haemodynamically stable (pulse down, BP rising and steady, warm peripheries, good urine output); 80% of bleeds stop spontaneously but 20% re-bleed.
7 Insert urinary catheter. Monitor urine output.
8 Consider inserting a CVP line, especially if the patient has a cardiac history or difficult venous access (consult your

senior). Keep CVP in the mid to normal range (there is a risk of a re-bleed if the pressure is kept too high).

Further investigations and ongoing medical management (discuss with your senior)

1 C&E. Bear in mind that urea is often raised due to blood in the gut, so look at the creatinine to assess renal status.
2 ECG and CXR in high risk patients. AXR is usually unhelpful in the acute setting.
3 Give IV ranitidine (50 mg tds) or equivalent. Switch to oral therapy as soon as possible, as it is much cheaper.
4 Monitor: pulse, BP, urine output (+/− CVP) hourly until stable. Slow the rate of transfusion once the pulse is less than 90 bpm and BP systolic is greater than 100 mmHg. Ask to be called if there are signs of:
  • Re-bleed.
  • Further haematemesis or malaena.
  • Pulse rate rises (by more than 10 bpm).
  • Systolic BP drops by more than 10 mmHg.
  • Urine output is less than 20 ml/hour.
  • The patient becomes confused.
5 Repeat clotting studies if patient has had more than 4 units transfused. You may need to give FFP (see p. 81).
6 Repeat FBC daily. Transfuse so that Hb > 10 g/dl.
7 Daily FBC and U, C&E. Repeat G&S if necessary (if previous sample used up).
8 Ensure 2 units of packed cells are

available for 48 hours after the bleeding has stopped.

9 Keep the patient NBM for 12 hours (longer if surgery is likely), and for at least 8 hours before endoscopy.

10 Ensure that the patient is on the next endoscopy list (usually the following morning) and that the endoscopist is informed. Obtain the patient's consent.

11 Consult with your team for further management.

Low risk patients

If after initial assessment the patient is well and at low risk of bleeding (e.g. only coffee-ground vomitus, no malaena, normal pulse, BP and JVP, warm peripheries):

• Take a history and examination to exclude the risk of a big bleed.

• Insert a cannula (just in case) and consider repeating a FBC and G&S.

• Inform your senior.

• Ask the nurses to monitor vital signs. Most patients will require no further action.

Hints

• Confirm with the patient that they have had true haematemesis, not haemoptysis or an occult nose-bleed.

• Vomitus can look like coffee grounds and contain small amounts of blood if the patient has not eaten for several days.

• In acute bleeds, the reported Hb lags approximately 12 hours behind the actual red cell loss. The *minimum* amount for transfusion is 1 U/g of Hb deficit; be guided by the clinical signs.

Lower gastrointestinal bleeds

Major lower GI bleeds, usually heralded by fresh or altered blood PR, are much less common in the hospital setting than upper GI bleeds, but can be just as serious. If called for a lower GI bleed, first exclude local causes such as piles and fissures and remember that major upper GI bleeds can present with altered blood PR. Follow the protocol for upper GI bleeds, with the possible addition of an urgent sigmoidoscopy. Discuss with your senior.

Glucose

You may be called for abnormal ward glucose readings. While *hyper*glycaemia is rarely an emergency, patients can die or suffer brain damage from *hypo*glycaemia, so need urgent attention.

On the ward

Hypoglycaemia is usually caused by oral hypoglycaemic agents, poor insulin control and faulty ward glucose readings:

1 See the patient. If they are alert and well, repeat the blood glucose stick and take a sample for an urgent glucose test from the laboratory. Give them a concentrated sugar drink, such as sweet tea, and some biscuits.

2 If the patient cannot drink or is unconscious, administer 50 ml of 50% dextrose IV immediately. Flush the vein

with 50 ml of saline, as concentrated dextrose is highly irritant. Also give 1 mg glucagon SC or IM.

3 Check the drug chart and recent insulin or oral hypoglycaemic doses. Adjust as necessary. Consider other, much rarer causes of hypoglycaemia in the hospital setting, including liver failure and acute alcohol consumption (which can and does occur in hospital).

4 Ask the nurse to repeat ward glucose readings. If the patient was semi-conscious or unconscious, repeat hourly until stable. Ask to be called if ward glucose readings are lower than 5 or more than 11 mmol/l.

5 If the patient overdosed on long-acting insulin or an oral hypoglycaemic agent, set up a 10% dextrose drip and adjust the rate according to blood glucose readings (4–6-hourly once fully conscious and readings normal). Keep the drip running for at least 48 hours.

Hyperglycaemia is commonly caused in diabetics by acute illness, corticosteroid treatment and test error. Hyperglycaemia in non-diabetics may be caused by blood being taken 'upstream' from a glucose-containing drip; from latent carbohydrate intolerance which may be unmasked by sepsis; acute stress (e.g. MI) and steroids; and from laboratory error. Do not overreact to mildly elevated blood glucose (e.g. 11 mmol/l) on a single occasion. DKA or hyper-osmolar complications take days to develop:

1 See the patient. Repeat the blood glucose stick and also send blood for urgent biochemistry glucose analysis. Make sure the sample is not taken from a 'drip' arm.

2 Check urinary ketones. If positive do ABGs and manage as for early DKA. If negative and the lab glucose result is greater than 22 mmol/l, give an immediate dose of insulin (5–10 U Actrapid SC) and discuss a diabetic regime with your senior.

3 If the patient is diabetic with consistently elevated blood glucose, consider changing their drug management.

Hints

• Laboratory glucose results are 10% higher and more accurate than finger-prick assays.
• NIDDM may require insulin for control during acute illness (see p. 185).

Gynaecological calls

Gynaecological problems should be considered when investigating common symptoms such as abdominal pain and anaemia. If you are confronted with a complex gynaecological or obstetric problem, do not hesitate to refer to the specialists.

Vaginal bleeding

Menstrual bleeding is common in hospital, but if the patient is post-menopausal or the bleeding abnormal, carcinoma of the cervix and uterus must be excluded.

Differential diagnoses
Menstrual bleeding (illness can cause abnormal periods)

continued

Break-through bleed on the oral contraceptive pill, especially if the patient is taking antibiotics
PID, especially if IUCD *in situ*
Fibroids or endometriosis
Tumours, especially cervical or uterine
Threatened miscarriage or ectopic pregnancy

On the ward

• Confirm that bleeding is vaginal and not rectal.
• Exclude pregnancy-related bleeding (ask about the LMP, contraceptive use and recent sexual history). Always think of pregnancy in pre-menopausal women. Send urine to the biochemistry lab for testing if the doubt.
• Consider PID, especially if low grade fever or tender abdomen. Do a PV examination for pelvic tenderness.
• Get a gynaecological referral if the patient is post-menopausal, or pre-

menopausal with persistent bleeding and no obvious cause.
• Investigations to consider:
   • Pap smear.
   • FBC, clotting studies, ESR/CRP.

Hint

• Anticoagulation does not cause abnormal PV bleeding but may unmask mucosal defects or tumours. Refer to a gynaecologist if the INR is within the therapeutic range.

Dysmenorrhoea

This is a common and painful problem for menstruating women.

On the ward

• Differentiate the pain from other causes of cramping, and lower abdominal pain. Most women will recognize period pain.
• Ask what medication works for

Table 7.6 Differential diagnoses of haematuria (consider the anatomy of the renal tract).

Renal tract	Extra-renal
• UTI • Trauma – catheters, surgery • Calculi • Prostatic disease • Tumours • Bladder inflammation (e.g. infection, recent surgery, chemotherapy)	*Systemic disorder* • Bleeding diathesis • Vasculitis (SLE, SBE etc.) • Malignant hypertension • Emboli • Sickle cell disease
Parenchymal disease • Acute glomerulonephritis • Cystic diseases • Tumours • Analgesic nephropathy • TB	

the patient and prescribe this if there is no contraindication. Mefenamic acid 500 mg tds or ibuprofen 400–600 mg tds are useful. The side effects and contraindications are the same as those for all NSAIDs. Co-proxamol or codeine are perfectly acceptable alternatives. A hot water bottle also helps.

Haematuria

In the hospital setting, haematuria is commonly caused by UTI or catheterization. However, haematuria may be the first sign of serious renal tract disease, such as tumour or renal parenchymal disease (see Table 7.6).

On the ward

1 Exclude vaginal or ano-rectal bleeding (common sources of false-positives.)
2 Test for UTI: scnd an MSU and repeat the dipstick (look for blood and protein). If symptomatic (dysuria, frequency +/− low grade fever) treat for UTI once the MSU is sent (see p. 99).
3 If a UTI is unlikely or the patient is unwell, discuss with your senior. Consider other causes (see above) and further investigations in light of clinical context:
  • Urine cytology.
  • FBC, ESR, CRP, C&E.
  • AXR for calculi; urogram.
  • Repeat urinary dipstick daily until diagnosis is clear.

Hints

• Urinary catheters can cause slight haematuria and usually do not require active treatment unless infection or non-trivial trauma is present.
• If the urinary dipstick reveals significant proteinuria (++ or more), renal parenchymal disease becomes more likely than a UTI. A very fresh sample of urine must be examined urgently for casts, etc. Commence a 24-hour urine collection to measure protein and creatinine clearance.
• If no red cells are seen on microscopy despite significant dipstick positive haematuria, consider haemolysis or myoglobinuria (rare).
• Anticoagulation within the therapeutic range rarely causes haematuria, but may unmask renal tract pathology. Repeat the clotting studies and discuss with your senior.

Headaches

Tension headaches are common in hospital. However, a severe headache with additional symptoms can be serious. The key to the diagnosis is the history.

Differential diagnoses and key symptoms

1 *Tension headache:* no associated symtoms Pain can be severe, usually symmetrical and band-like.
2 *Migraine:* usually history of previous episodes. Severe, throbbing pain which may be unilateral or asymmetric. May have prodromal symptoms (visual symptoms such as flashing lights, tunnel vision, cranial nerve deficit rarely lasting more than 1 hour, N&V, photophobia). Classic history makes the diagnosis, but exclude other causes if drowsy, neuro-

continued

logical deficit or visual symptoms. A variant is *cluster headaches*: unilateral pain becomes severe around one eye which becomes red, swollen and watery. Episodes last up to 1 hour, and can occur several times a day.

3 *Sinusitis:* dull, unilateral or central frontal headache. Local tenderness.

4 *Drug-induced:* especially nitrates, digoxin, tricyclic antidepressants, benzodiazepines (the morning after).

5 *Meningitis, encephalitis:* photophobia, stiff neck, +/- fever and rash. Requires urgent LP (if no signs of raised ICP or focal neurology) and antibiotics.

6 *Subarachnoid haemorrhage:* sudden onset of severe headache (like an explosion in the head) and meningism. Occasional atypical history (small leaks) mimicking meningitis. CT scan +/- LP (showing red cells uniformly spread throughout the CSF).

7 *Raised ICP:* present on waking, often associated vomiting. May have blurred vision, raised BP, slow pulse.

8 *Brain abscess:* non-specific pain. Diagnosis requires index of suspicion and CT scan.

9 *Hypertensive encephalopathy:* always markedly elevated BP (diastolic >130 mmHg) and other signs of malignant hypertension (p. 66).

10 *Subdural haematoma:* elderly, alcoholic, head trauma.

11 *Acute glaucoma:* usually presents with a dull pain behind the eyes which the patient may describe as a headache. Early: mildly injected conjuctiva. Later: overtly red eyes. Urgent ophthalmology referral required.

12 *Temporal arteritis:* patient >50 years old. Subacute onset of frontal headache. Commonly associated with fever, malaise, myalgia, weight loss, unilateral blindness or other visual disturbance (indicating imminent occlusion of the ophthalmic artery). A typical history, tender temporal arteries and a markedly raised ESR establish the diagnosis. Temporal artery biopsy may be negative.

On the ward

1 See the patient. Briefly exclude emergencies (meningitis, encephalitis, subdural haematoma, subarachnoid haemaorrhage, acute glaucoma, temporal arteritis) with symptoms and signs (see box above).

2 Do a history and examination. Ask the patient if they have had similar headaches before (consider tension headaches, migraine and sinusitis). If history is typical for tension headache or migraine, and there is no evidence of fever, neck-stiffness, raised ICP, or temporal artery tenderness, prescribe analgesia (see below). However, if the headache is persistent, you should examine:

• Pupils and fundi (raised ICP).
• ENT (otitis media, sinusitis).
• CNS (especially cranial nerves).
• Gait (if history suggestive of space occupying lesion).
• Palpate temporal arteries for tenderness.

3 Investigations to consider:
If the history is typical for a tension headache or migraine, and there are no sinister signs, then no investigations are necessary. Otherwise consider (depending on clinical context):

- ESR, CRP.
- LP and CT scan, sinus X-ray.
- Temporal artery biopsy, but a negative result does not exclude skip lesions.

4 Treatment:

Once the rare but serious causes are excluded, 1 g of paracetamol 4–6-hourly prn is usually effective. If the patient is already on paracetamol, try ibuprofen (400–600 mg qds) unless NSAIDs are contraindicated. The next line of therapy is codeine phosphate or equivalent. If sub-occipital or cervical muscle spasm is present, cyclobenzaprine 10 mg tds (a muscle relaxant) may be effective.

Hints

- Always consider meningitis in patients with fever and headache, although any febrile illness may have an associated throbbing headache.
- The scalp may be tender with tension headaches, migraine, temporal arteritis or shingles.
- Be alert to depression in patients with recurrent tension headaches or migraines.

Hypertension

Hypertension is common but rarely requires treatment in the middle of the night unless there is evidence of heart failure, malignant hypertension, or severe renal disease.

On the ward

1 Re-check BP and pulse. Note previous readings. Make sure you use a big enough manometer cuff if the patient has large arms.

2 Exclude:
- Heart failure: raised JVP, basal crackles, swollen ankles, enlarged liver.
- Malignant hypertension: headache; confusion or depressed level of consciousness; deteriorating vision. Perform fundoscopy to check for fresh retinal haemorrhages, and dipstick urine for haematuria/proteinuria.
- Renal failure: check urine output and recent creatinine result.

If heart failure, malignant hypertension or renal failure, start to treat the cause and call the medical registrar for further management.

3 Otherwise, an elevated BP alone is seldom an indication for treatment. However, if the diastolic BP is greater than 130 mmHg, put the patient to bed and prescribe an oral beta-blocker (if no contraindication) or a calcium channel blocker and aim to reduce the blood pressure slowly over 2–3 days. SL nifedipine can cause a dramatic fall in BP, so do not use without consulting your firm's policy. Call your senior if there is no response within 1 hour.

4 If the patient is in pain or very anxious (common causes of elevated systolic pressure), provide analgesia and reassurance as appropriate.

Peri-op hypertension (see also Surgery, p. 181)

Pre-op hypertension: Most anaesthetists will not anaesthetize a patient with a diastolic BP > 100 mmHg. Discuss prescribing 10 mg of nifedipine PO or further sedation with the anaesthetist or your senior. 5 mg SL nifedipine will reduce the blood pressure within 5 minutes and may be repeated. Ensure the anaesthetist is aware of the problem.

Post-op hypertension is often related to pain and will settle with adequate analgesia. If persistent, discuss with your senior.

Hints

• Do not treat hypertension for at least 48 hours following a CVA. Dropping the BP under these circumstances can cause brain damage.
• Raised ICP can cause hypertension and bradycardia (Cushings reflex).

Hypotension

Hypotension is a common call, particularly post-op. Hypotension is seldom an emergency, but while on the phone ask how far the BP has fallen. A fall in systolic BP of > 20 mmHg is significant and > 40 mmHg (or systolic BP < 80 mmHg) is an emergency (see The moribund patient p. 70).

Differential diagnoses
Low blood volume (bleeding, dehydration)
Low peripheral resistance (post-general anaesthetic, infection, vaso–vagal, drugs: ACE inhibitors, nitrates, antihypertensives)
Failing heart (arrhythmia, CCF)

On the ward

1 See the patient and repeat the BP. If well but feeling faint, vaso–vagal or drug

causes (including general anaesthesia) are likely. Drop the patient's head and raise their legs. Check the drug chart and do an ECG. Observe.

2 If unwell, feel their peripheries. If the patient has cold, clammy peripheries, consider:
• Hypovolaemia (bleeding or dehydrated: JVP down).
• Cardiac causes (MI, arrhythmia: raised JVP. Check for irregular pulse, basal crepitations, history of IHD, chest pain).
• PE (raised JVP, short of breath. Check legs for DVT, often no specific signs).
• Anaphylaxis (wheezy, short of breath, new drug started).

If the patient has warm peripheries, consider:
• Sepsis (JVP variable, fever). Check for source of infection (chest, abdomen, urine, skin, cannulae, surgical wounds). Exclude immunocompromise (see p. 56). Note that in some patients, severe sepsis may cause circulatory shutdown (cold peripheries) without going through a stage of vasodilatation.

3 Treat according to the cause. If hypovolaemic:
• Place the patient's head down.
• Insert large bore IV cannulae. Give rapid IV fluid (e.g. Haemaccel)
• Face-mask O_2 100% (at least in the short term).
• Catheterize and monitor urine output.
• Consult your senior.

If cardiac causes are most likely:
• The patient may go into shock. Get senior help and do an ECG stat.
• Give face-mask O_2 100% (at least in the short term).

- Sit the patient up if it is more comfortable for them.
- Arrange for a mobile CXR.

If septic:
- Large bore IV access, rapid IV fluids.
- Face-mask O₂ 100%.
- Blood cultures (two times) are mandatory, FBC, C&E.
- Consult your senior urgently before giving broad spectrum antibiotic cover.

Less common causes:
- PE. Do urgent ECG, CXR and ABGs. Discuss anticoagulation with your senior.
- Anaphylaxis. Give 100% O₂; adrenaline 1 ml of a 1:1000 solution IM/IV; salbutamol 5 mg nebulizer if wheezy; hydrocortisone 100 mg IV and chlorpheniramine 10 mg IV.
- Consider adrenal insufficiency, especially if the patient is on steroids or has a history of Addisons. Give hydrocortisone 100 mg IV (to cover the added stress of illness irrespective of the cause).

4 If you feel out of your depth, call for senior help immediately. Most often the cause is obvious but if not, do the following until help arrives:
- IV access.
- Face-mask O₂.
- ECG and mobile CXR.
- Bloods: FBC and clotting screen (INR and APTT); C&E; glucose; G&S (cross-match if suspect bleeding—see GI bleeds p. 59); ABGs or at least pulse oximeter, and blood cultures.
- Monitor urine output and consider catheterization.

Hints

- Post-op falls in BP are common and often due to opiate analgesia. If the patient is otherwise well with no evidence of bleeding, ask the nurses to continue to monitor the T, BP and pulse and to call you if the patient becomes unwell or the BP substantially dips from its post-op plateau. The BP should rise as the anaesthesia wears off.
- Always re-check the BP yourself, remembering to use a big enough cuff for large arms.
- Bradycardia suggests a vaso-vagal or arrhythmia (e.g. complete heart block unless the patient is on beta-blockers or has raised ICP).
- If the patient is hypovolaemic, but there is no evidence of dehydration or bleeding, consider an occult bleed. Risk factors for occult bleeding include NSAIDs, stress ulceration, recent instrumentation/surgery, hidden fractures (especially in the elderly).
- Dehydration is common in frail patients.

Insomnia

Avoid prescribing sleeping tablets without first considering why the patient can't sleep. Having said that, it can be very difficult to sleep on a ward, and providing the patient does not take them home, short-acting sleeping tablets can be very helpful.

Differential diagnosis and suggested management:

1 **Noise, light or too much daytime sleep.** These are the commonest causes of insomnia in hospital and often the

hardest to fix. Common sense suggestions include:

- Suggesting that the patient need not worry about not sleeping at night. If they really need to sleep, they will.
- Avoiding stimulants before bedtime, such as cigarettes, tea or coffee.
- Wearing ear plugs and an eye visor at night.
- Ask the nursing staff whether it is possible to cancel the patient's early morning observations. Minimize noise from monitors. Resolve conflicts between patients (consider moving beds around).
- Move the patient to a side room if possible, or to a quieter corner of the ward.

2 **Pain:**
- Analgesia will facilitate sleep better than sleeping tablets.

3 **Confusion, excessive anxiety or irritation, depression:**
- Do not sedate the patient without excluding medical causes such as hypoxia, alcohol withdrawal, wrong drug dosages or electrolyte derangements (check fluid and drug charts).
- Depression is common in hospital patients (see p. 106). Be wary of inducing benzodiazepine addiction in such patients (who may be especially vulnerable). Seek psychiatric and pharmacological advice if in doubt.

4 **Disturbed sleep pattern due to frequency of micturition, orthopnoea or PND.**
- The patient may need better control of LVF. Avoid prescribing diuretics close to bedtime.

5 **Disturbance in regular medication and bedtime habits:**

- Often patients take an over-the-counter 'sleeping remedy' at home or have a supply of sleeping tablets which are not included in the GP's letter. The patient may not inform you about them unless specifically asked, and may suffer rebound insomnia in hospital.
- You can prescribe patients a tot or two of liquor before bedtime if they are used to it—but ask your senior first!

Management with benzodiazepines

Benzodiazepines (e.g. Temazepam 10–20 mg or Oxazepam 15–30 mg) are the mainstay of therapy for insomnia but some patients cannot tolerate them. A useful alternative is chloral hydrate (500–1000 mg PO or PR) but do not use in patients with renal or hepatic failure. Amitriptyline 25–50 mg nocte is useful when chronic pain accompanies sleep disturbance. Use lower doses of all sedatives in the elderly (consult the *BNF*).

- If you prescribe a sedative, tell the patient to call the nursing staff if they need the toilet. Sedatives in an unfamiliar environment can cause falls.

Itching

Except in the unusual event of anaphylaxis, itching is rarely serious, but can be very distressing for the patient. Exclude simple dermatological problems before considering symptomatic treatment if the patient has skin lesions or a rash (see Rashes pp. 76–77).

Differential diagnoses (if no visible skin lesions or rash)
• Dry skin
• Drugs or allergies
• Jaundice
• Early shingles
• Infestations (scabies, lice)
• Rarities: Polycythaemia rubra vera
            (myeloproliferative
            diseases)
            Hodgkin's lymphoma
            Late renal failure

On the ward

1 Check the patient's skin for rashes or lesions. If present see Rashes pp. 76–77.
2 If there are no visible skin lesions, by far the most common cause of itching is dry skin, followed by drug reactions. Try to identify and replace the drug (seek pharmacological advice if unsure). Treat with emollient lotions after bathing (e.g. Calamine Lotion). Use cold compresses and moisturizers such as E-45 for localized itching. Advise minimal use of soap and shampoo. Discuss alternatives with nurses.
3 If you are called at night and the patient is well, it is reasonable to treat symptomatically. Choose a sedating antihistamine at night (e.g. chlorpheniramine 4 mg tds) or a non-sedating one if preferred by the patient (e.g. terfenadine 60 mg bd).

Hint

• Scabies is common and can cause intense itching anywhere on the body except the head. The S-shaped burrows are easy to miss—look carefully around the itching site, particularly along the

fingers and in the webs. Contrary to popular mythology, scabies does not imply that the patient is unhygienic! Consult the *BNF* for treatment of scabies and other infestations. Clothes and bedding need to be washed.

The moribund patient

If you are called to see a 'flat' patient, don't panic. You usually have more time than you think. The priority is to buy time by supporting the vital functions while getting basic background information and examining as you go. Call your senior early and don't be afraid to call the crash team *before* the patient arrests. Think CASH (Table 7.7)!

On the ward

1 See the patient urgently. Check their ABC:

Airway clear?	Y/N
Breathing?	Y/N
	Trachea central?
	Bilateral breath sounds?
Circulation?	Pulse? – Y/N
	If Y – BP?

2 Establish large bore IV access: 16 G (grey) if possible. Don't rush. Consider inserting two cannulae at separate sites.
3 Give O_2.
4 If BP < 80 mmHg, consider starting a rapid colloid infusion (Haemaccel) unless a cardiac cause is probable. Use saline if sepsis is likely.
5 While the infusion is being set up, quickly assess preceding symptoms, PMH and current medications. Examine the chest and heart.
6 If a cardiac cause is likely:

• Do an ECG and request a mobile CXR. Do not delay treatment.
• Pulmonary oedema, arrhythmias or MI are the most likely causes. Consider pericardial tamponade.

7 Exclude hypoglycaemia or opiate overdose:
• If blood glucose is less than 2.5 mmol/l, give 50 ml of 50% glucose IV (flush vein with saline afterwards) or 1 mg glucagon IV/IM/SC.
• Note the size of pupils. Give naloxone 400–800 μg IV if the patient has pinpoint pupils and is on opiates. Repeat if necessary.

8 Listen to the chest. If markedly tachypnoeic in the absence of pulmonary oedema or pneumothorax, consider PE.

9 Feel the peripheries. If the patient has warm peripheries with hypotension, consider sepsis.

10 Consider anaphylaxis:
• New drug started recently, hypotensive, SOB, wheezy, swollen lips/eyelids, urticarial rash.
• Give 100% O_2; adrenaline 1 ml of a 1 : 1000 solution IM/IV; salbutamol 5 mg nebulizer; hydrocortisone 100 mg IV and chlorpheniramine 10 mg IV.

If the cause is not clear, do a brief neurological examination: level of consciousness (obeying commands), pupils and eye movements, limb tone, reflexes and plantars. Consider occult bleeding. Seek senior advice.

11 Urgent investigations:
• ECG.
• FBC and INR, C&E, glucose, amylase.
• ABGs.
• Mobile CXR, as erect as possible to check for free air under the diaphragm. View carefully for a pneumothorax, often missed in a panic.

Hints

• Metabolic acidosis, confirmed by an ABG, can cause tachypnoea. If the patient has metabolic acidosis and hypotension consider sepsis, ischaemic bowel or perforated viscus or pancreatitis and acute renal failure.
• Relieve a tension pneumothorax by inserting a needle or Venflon into the

Table 7.7 Differential diagnoses. (Acronym: CASH.)

Chest	Abdomen	Systemic	Head
Pulmonary oedema MI, arrhythmia Pneumonia Asthma Pulmonary embolus Dissecting aneurysm Tension pneumothorax	Haemorrhage Perforated viscus Pancreatitis	Durg overdose, especially opiates Hypothermia Septicaemia Hypoglycaemia Anaphylaxis Serious electrolyte derangement or dehydration	CVA Post-ictal

second intercostal space, mid-clavicular line.

Nausea and vomiting

Any acute illness can cause non-specific N&V. However, be wary of prescribing anti-emetics without also investigating the cause if the patient is distressed it is reasonable to give an anti-emetic before examining them.

Differential diagnoses
1 Surgical conditions
Intestinal obstruction (adhesion, hernias, tumours) and Peritonism (perforation, pancreatitis etc.)

2 Medical causes
Local causes
Oesophagitis
Gastritis
Peptic ulcer

Central causes
Raised ICP (tumour, meningitis, subdural etc.)
Migraine

Systemic causes
Infection (UTI, pneumonia, gastroenteritis)
Metabolic (organ failure, electrolyte imbalance—Na, K, Ca)
Drug reactions (opiates, digoxin, NSAIDs, dopamine agonists, chemotherapy)

3 Special causes
Pregnancy
Inferior acute MI

On the ward

1 Exclude severe dehydration (BP sitting and lying).
2 Rule out common surgical conditions—**Intestinal obstruction** and **peritonism**.
3 Think about **medical causes** as above.
4 **Special considerations:**
  (a) Is the patient pregnant? Do βHCG
  (b) In the elderly, an inferior acute MI can present with N&V in the absence of pain. Do ECG and serial cardiac enzymes.
5 When there is **no obvious cause** after history and examination
  (a) If the patient had a single episode of vomiting without associated symptoms or signs, ask the nurses to observe the patient and monitor T, BP, pulse and urine output. Dipstick the urine
  (b) If the patient has persistent N&V or systemic upset, consider:
  (c) MSU, FBC, C&E.
6 Further investigations to consider include:
  • Ca, Mg, phosphate, amylase.
  • ABGs if severe vomiting.
7 Management options to control symptoms:
The two most commonly used drugs are prochlorperazine: 25 mg PR or 12.5 mg IM and metoclopramide 10 mg IM or IV (caution in young women for dystonic reactions). Alternatives include:
  • Cyclizine lactate: 50 mg IM or IV.
  • Domperidone: 30–60 mg PR.

• Droperidol: 1–10 mg IV or IM.
• 5-HT$_3$ antagonists (e.g. ondansetron, granisetron) are very effective but are expensive and usually reserved for chemotherapy-induced N&V.
• Diphenhydramine counteracts extra-pyramidal side effects of phenothiazines.

Oxygen therapy

This section describes how to give O$_2$ safely, particularly to patients with COAD.

Methods of oxygen delivery

Face-masks (e.g. system 22 or Ventimasks) are good for the acute situation but can be replaced with nasal specs (see below) for longer term use. *Controlled percentage* face masks control the amount of O$_2$ the patient recieves, and are graded 24%, 28%, 35%, 40% and 60%. You need to adjust the O$_2$ flow rate at the wall or cylinder, according to the rate printed on the mask—usually about 2 litres/minute for 24% masks and 15 litres/minute for 60% masks. It takes at least 15–20 minutes for blood gases to equilibrate after changing the percentage of inspired O$_2$.

Nasal specs are useful if the patient cannot tolerate a face-mask and for longer-term O$_2$ therapy. It is difficult to regulate O$_2$ delivery with nasal specs so regular blood gas checks may be necessary. For standard size specs, a flow rate of 4–6 litres/minute is usual for achieving an inspired O$_2$ percentage of 30–40%.

For patients with chronic obstructive airways disease

Under normal conditions, the concentration of CO$_2$ in the blood is the primary stimulus of the respiratory drive. Some patients with severe COAD become insensitive to CO$_2$ levels and are dependent on low O$_2$ levels (mild hypoxia) to maintain their respiratory effort. If you give too much O$_2$ the hypoxic stimulus is lost and they will hypoventilate leading to CO$_2$ retention (hypercarbia). This can lead to CO$_2$ narcosis and death.

Therefore, when *non-emergency* O$_2$ therapy is required in patients with COAD:
1 Start with a 24% face-mask and measure the ABGs after 1 hour to ensure that the CO$_2$ levels are not rising. You need to find a level that achieves a fine balance between improving oxygenation and keeping the CO$_2$ at a safe level. Ask for senior advice if the CO$_2$ level rises >1.5 kPa above the previous ABG level or rises above 8 kPa.
2 If the CO$_2$ level does not rise but hypoxia is still a problem, increase the oxygen to 28% then 35% etc., repeating the ABGs an hour after each change.
3 If you cannot increase the percentage O$_2$, despite persisting hypoxia, because of hypercarbia, a doxapram infusion or mechanical ventilation may be necessary—discuss with your team.

In emergencies, use *100% O$_2$, even when the patient is known to have moderately severe COAD (unless you

---

* In practice, unrestricted use of an ordinary (non-anaesthetic) face-mask will only deliver about 60% O$_2$.

know they are fitting from CO_2 narcosis!). Hypoxia kills quickly (within minutes) whereas CO_2 narcosis kills slowly (over hours). You will have time to check the ABGs if there is a history of COAD.

Hints

- Use a humidifier with O_2 if possible.
- Patients may be left on O_2 for longer than they need it. Always ask whether or not they really need it. The face-mask and straps are uncomfortable and can cause nasty abrasions and bruises to the face of patients on warfarin or steroids.
- Strictly, you are supposed to prescribe O_2 therapy on the drug chart.

Pulse oximetry

Pulse oximetry measures the percentage of blood O_2 saturation, and is not a direct assay of Pao_2 or $Paco_2$. It is not as trustworthy as arterial blood gases, particularly in COAD patients, as they may retain CO_2 in spite of reasonable percentage O_2 saturation. Also, pulse oximetry will not reveal quite a low Pao_2. Remember that the O_2 saturation curve for Hb is a steep sigmoid curve that starts to plateau around a Pao_2 of 9.1 kPa (70 mmHg). This means a patient may have a very low Pao_2 of 8.5 kPa and still have better than 90% O_2 saturation. If in doubt do ABGs.

Phlebitis

Phlebitis is indicated by pain and redness at IV sites, and is prevented by changing the IV site every 2–3 days (important if the patient has a cardiac valve lesion or prosthetic valve).

Management

1 Remove the cannula and apply heat (e.g. damp, warm towel).
2 Elevate the limb.
3 Give mild analgesia if the site is very painful (e.g. a NSAID such as ibuprofen 400–600 mg tds).
4 Suppurative phlebitis is more worrying (pus at the IV entry site, induration, fever and enlarged draining lymph nodes). Try to express some pus and send a swab to microbiology for urgent MC&S. Prescribe IV antibiotics to cover *Staphylococcus aureus*. If the patient is well, flucloxacillin alone may suffice. Discuss local protocols with a microbiologist. Surgical drainage is sometimes required.

Potassium

Hyperkalaemia

K greater than 6.5 mmol/l needs urgent treatment, but first exclude false positives from old samples. Repeat the sample if in doubt. In the hospital setting, by far the commonest cause of hyperkalaemia is drugs.

Differential diagnoses
Drugs
K sparing diuretics – spironolactone, amiloride, triamterene
ACE inhibitors
Excessive K supplements

continued

Metabolic acidosis
Acute renal failure
Diabetic ketoacidosis

Cell lysis
Massive tissue trauma
Massive blood transfusion

Mineralocorticoid deficiency
Addison's disease

On the ward

1 See the patient. Repeat K and check their renal function (U, C&E). In the meantime, if the initial K was greater than 6.5:

2 Do an ECG urgently (look for widened QRS complexes and peaked T waves).

3 Give calcium gluconate 10 ml of a 10% solution IV over 10 minutes.

4 Do urgent ABGs. If acidotic, discuss with your senior. The use of bicarbonate (100 ml of a 4.2% solution) is highly controversial.

5 Give 10–15 units soluble insulin with 50 g of glucose 50% IV.

6 Set up a continuous 50% glc infusion (50 ml/hour) with insulin according to 1–2-hourly glucose readings (insulin drives K back into cells).

7 Consider polystyrene sulphonate resin (Ca resonium) 15 g 6–8-hourly PO or 30 g in methylcellulose solution PR. As this causes severe constipation, consider giving a laxative at the same time.

Hypokalaemia

In the hospital setting, hypokalaemia is usually caused by diuretics, in-

appropiate replacement fluids or taking blood from the drip arm.

Differential diagnoses
Inadequate potassium replacement in IV fluids

Renal losses
Diuretics
Other drugs—amphotericin B, carbenicillin, ticarcillin
Excess mineralocorticoid (tumours)

GIT losses
Diarrhoea
Vomiting
Intestinal fistulae, villous adenoma

Intracellular potassium shifts
Alkalosis
Insulin and glucose administration

On the ward

1 See the patient. If the K is less than 2.5 mmol/l, or less than 3.0 *and* the patient is taking digoxin, you need to replace K urgently, as there is a risk of arrhythmias:

• Give 20 mmol/hour KCl at a concentration not exceeding 40 mmol/l (60 mmol/l in emergencies). Concentrated K damages peripheral veins. Never give bolus KCl, which can cause fatal arrhythmias. If a central line is available, 20 mmol/hour in 50–100 ml of 5% dextrose can be infused, but ensure that the infusion rate is monitored.

• Do an urgent ECG, looking for low, small T-waves. Consider an ECG monitor. Patients with arrhythmias should be transferred to the CCU.

- Monitor K 4-hourly until stable.

2 If the K is between 2.5 and 3.0 mmol/l:
  - Oral replacement therapy is usually sufficient (see below). However, if the patient is at risk for arrhythmias (e.g. recent MI or on therapy for arrhythmias), give cautious IV therapy (10–15 mmol/hour).

3 If the K is greater than 3.0 mmol/l:
  - Give oral replacement therapy unless the patient is NBM or vomiting. Prescribe 80–120 mmol K in divided doses per day. There is a wide range of pills with varying amounts of K in each (see below). You can also advise the patient to eat K-containing foods such as bananas and chocolate.

4 Investigations to consider:
  - Monitor K every 1–2 days.
  - Do ABGs if you suspect alkalosis (alkalosis causes intracellular K shifts).
  - Consider measuring Mg. Hypomagnesaemia is a common problem when hypokalaemia is due to chronic renal losses and may cause the hypokalaemia to be refractory to therapy.

A rough guide to calculating the total amount of potassium replacement required

In adults, a drop of plasma K from 4 to 3 mmol/l represents a total body deficit of 100–200 mmol K (depending on body weight). Each further 1 mmol/l drop below 3 mmol/l represents a deficit of an additional 200–400 mmol K.

Oral replacement therapy

K content of oral supplements:

- Slow-K   8 mmol K (effervescent)
- Sando-K   12 mmol K (tablet)
- Kay-Cee-L   1 mmol/ml (syrup, if the patient won't take tablets)

Hints

- Avoid Slow-K non-effervescent tablets, as they cause severe oesophageal and gastric irritation. Use the horrible tasting, but more effective, soluble effervescent tablets or syrups.
- In patients with normal renal function, it is difficult to overdose with oral K. However, DO NOT give K if the patient is oliguric. Consult your senior.
- Low plasma bicarbonate levels suggest that the patient has long-standing, intracellular K depletion. K replacement can take days.
- Contrary to popular belief, hypokalaemia secondary to vomiting is due to metabolic alkalosis (which causes intracellular K shift and renal excretion of K), not to loss of K in gastric juices, which contain very little K.
- Be careful in prescribing long-term oral K supplements for patients to take home. Make sure that the GP knows to monitor the patient's K, to avoid hyperkalaemia.

Rashes and skin lesions

The algorithm below is designed to help you make an initial diagnosis of your patient's rash or skin lesion. By far the commonest cause of new rashes in hospital is drug reactions, but psoriasis, shingles and other relapsing skin conditions can all flare up with the stress of illness. Dermatologists are usually very helpful and keen for referrals. Seek their help if in any doubt. Questions to ask are:

1 Are the lesions filled with fluid?
   No – go to the next question.
   Clear fluid   (1) vesiculobullous
                      diseases.
   Pus   (2) pustular diseases.
2 Are the lesions coloured but not red?
   Yellow   (3) yellow lesions.
   White   (4) white lesions.
   Brown   (5) brown lesions.
   Skin coloured (6) skin coloured
                      papules and
                      nodules.
3 If the lesions are red, are they scaling?
   No scaling:
   Macular/flat   (7) vascular reactions.
   Papular/   (8) inflammatory
   raised   papules/nodules.
   Scaling:
   No epithelial (9) papulosquamous
     disruption   diseases.
   Epithelial   (10) eczematous
     disruption   reactions.

Disease categories (1)–(10)

1 **Vesiculobullous diseases:**
   • Vesicles: Herpes simplex; shingles; chicken pox; tinea pedis; scabies; dermatitis herpetiformis; dyshidrosis.
   • Bullae: pemphigus; pemphigoid; bullous impetigo; erythema multiforme bullosum.
2 **Pustular diseases:**
   • Acne; folliculitis; candidiasis; rosacea.
3 **Yellow lesions:**
   • Xanthelasma; necrobiosis lipoidicum.

4 **White lesions:**
   • Tinea versicolor; pityriasis alba; vitiligo.
5 **Brown lesions:**
   • Macules – freckles and lentigenes.
   • Papules and nodules – junctional or compound naevi; melanoma; seborrhoeic keratoses.
   • Patches and plaques – café-au-lait spots; giant pigmented hairy naevus.
6 **Skin coloured papules and nodules:**
   • Rough surface – warts; actinic keratoses; squamous cell carcinoma.
   • Smooth surface – condylomata acuminata; basal cell carcinoma; epidermoid cysts; lipomas; molluscum contagiosum.
7 **Vascular reactions:**
   • Blanching lesions – macular and diffuse erythema (toxic erythema, e.g. skin rash of viral illness); urticaria; erythema multiforme; erythema nodosum.
   • Non-blanching (purpuric) lesions – the vasculitides.
8 **Inflammatory papules and nodules:**
   • Papules – insect bites; pyogenic granulomas; cherry angiomas; granuloma annulare.
   • Nodules – furunculosis +/− cellulitis.
9 **Papulosquamous diseases:**
   • Plaque formation – psoriasis; lupus erythematosus; mycosis fungoides; tinea corporis; tinea cruris and tinea pedis.
   • Predominantly papular – lichen planus, secondary syphilis, pityriasis rosea.
10 **Eczematous reactions:**
   • Atopic dermatitis; dyshidrotic eczema; contact dermatitis; others.

Diagnosing skin tumours

Melanoma
Itching; crusting; bleeding; change in size, shape or colour of mole; weight loss; satellite lesions

Basal cell carcinoma
Pearly nodule/ulcer with prominent blood vessels

Squamous cell carcinoma
Non-healing; crusting ulcer with rolled edge

Hint

• Generalized erythematous rash (+/− blistering) and fever should ring alarm bells as they may be associated with serious bacterial infections (e.g. streptococcal and staphylococcal).

Shortness of breath

When answering your bleep

• Ask the nurse to assess the respiratory rate, pulse, BP and, if possible, peak flows and pulse oximetry readings.

Differential diagnoses
Acute LVF
Asthma
Pulmonary embolus
Pneumonia
Pneumothorax
COAD exacerbated by acute illness

Rarely
Pericardial tamponade
Anaphylaxis

On the ward

1 See the patient. Check the T, BP and pulse and assess for respiratory distress (respiratory rate >30/minute +/− cyanosis) and hypotension.

2 If the patient is hypotensive, consider: acute MI, large PE, tension pneumothorax, pericardial tamponade and anaphylaxis. Lower the patient's head and institute emergency treatment. Get senior assistance (see Hypotension p. 67).

3 If the patient is markedly tachypnoeic or cyanosed:

• Give O_2. Even if the patient has COAD, it is safe to give initial O_2 and reduce as soon as possible (hypoxia kills quickly, high CO_2 kills slowly) (see p. 72).

• Exclude pneumothorax with auscultation.

• Give salbutamol 5 mg stat using a nebulizer. Repeat as necessary.

• Examine quickly for acute pulmonary oedema (JVP, basal crackles or effusion). If present, give frusemide 40 mg IV, diamorphine 5 mg IV slowly and an anti-emetic (e.g. metaclopramide 10 mg IV/IM). Consider MI or arrhythmia and do an urgent ECG.

• Request a mobile CXR.

• Do ABGs.

• Notify your senior. Get help early if the patient is deteriorating.

Important note: if you cannot distinguish between early pulmonary oedema, asthma or pneumonia (often difficult to differentiate), treat for all three (see [3] above). If there are no signs of heart failure or asthma, consider pulmonary embolus. Heparinize if in doubt (see p. 100) and confirm the diagnosis later.

4 If the patient is not acutely distressed: take a full history and examination. Don't forget to ask about chest pain or leg swelling, history of asthma or IHD, and any recent changes in medication. Consider the differential diagnosis and treat accordingly.

5 Investigations to consider:
  • FBC, C&E.
  • ABGs.
  • CXR (expiratory to show a pneumothorax better).
  • ECG.
  • Consider urgent ECHO if you suspect tamponade.

Hints

• Hypoxia can cause euphoria, so don't be reassured by an apparently undistressed patient. Be guided by the signs.
• A good way to assess respiratory rate is to breathe with the patient, as this also reveals abnormal breathing rhythms (not all dyspnoeic patients are tachypnoeic).
• Patients at risk for pneumothorax include those with a central line, pneumonia, COAD or asthma. Pneumothorax is easy to miss on CXR; ask for an expiratory film.
• Psychogenic SOB (hyperventilation) is suggested by peri-oral tingling, pins and needles, carpo-pedal spasm and especially alkalosis on ABGs. Treat by having the patient breathe into a paper bag.
• A fever suggests infection, but also consider PE or MI.
• Check for pulsus paradoxus (drop in BP of greater than 10 mmHg on inspiration), which suggests an acute exacerbation of COAD, asthma, or tamponade.
• If possible, take an ABG sample before starting the patient on O_2.

Diagnosing the important common conditions causing acute SOB

Acute LVF
Raised JVP
S3 gallop
Cold peripheries
Basal inspiratory crackles

Severe asthma
Pulse >120/minute, rate >30/minute
Pulsus paradoxus (BP drop >10 mmHg on inspiration)
PEFR <100
Rising $Paco_2$ (anything over 5 kPa is worrying in the face of tachypnoea)
Exhausted patient barely able to speak

Pulmonary embolus
DVT, pleuritic chest pain, pleural rub
RV strain: raised JVP, RV gallop
RV strain on ECG: prominent R waves in V1–V2 (common), inverted T waves in III and V1–4, deep S wave in I, Q wave in III (less common)

Pneumothorax
Chest hyper-resonant to percussion
Markedly decreased vocal resonance (a very useful sign!)
Decreased breath sounds
Often funny noises or clicks with heart beat during respiration

The sick patient

The following is a checklist of things that you should consider when seeing any patient who is very unwell (modify in light of the specific system involved):
1 What are the T, BP, pulse, respiratory rate?
2 Are ABC adequate?
3 Does the patient need:
  • Analgesia?
  • ABGs or pulse oximetry?
  • Baseline bloods?
  • CXR (mobile)?
  • ECG or ECG monitor?
  • IV access?
  • IV fluids?
  • O_2
  • Senior opinion?
  • Urinary catheter?

Sodium

Hyponatraemia

Mild to moderate hyponatraemia is common in hospital due to excess IV (hypotonic) fluids. Hyponatraemia usually develops over days; replacement of Na should be cautious. More urgent treatment is required if there are neurological symptoms which range from lethargy to severe confusion or coma, but symptoms should not be ascribed to hyponatraemia if the serum Na is >125 mmol/l.

Differential diagnoses
Over-hydration with IV fluids

Renal
Thiazide diuretics

Nephrotic syndrome
Addison's Disease
Interstitial renal disease

SIADH
Malignancy
CNS
Drugs – chlorpropamide, cytotoxics, haloperidol, thioridazine
Pus in the chest
Porphyria

Others
Cirrhosis
CCF
Severe hypothyroidism
Following relief of small bowel obstruction

On the ward

1 See the patient and assess their fluid balance (JVP, fluid chart, chest).
  • If dehydrated, measure urinary Na. If urinary Na >20 mmol/l with hyponatraemia, consider renal causes. If urinary Na <20 mmol/l consider other causes.
  • If not dehydrated, is the patient puffy?
  If yes, volume overload is likely but exclude nephrotic syndrome, CCF, cirrhosis and severe hypothyroidism. If no, but the urine is concentrated (osmolality >500 mmol/kg or high specific gravity), SIADH is most likely. Look for the cause (see above).
2 Investigations to consider:
  • Urinary Na, urine and plasma osmolality, U&E, liver chemistry.
  • CXR.
  • Discuss others with senior according to clinical setting.
3 Management: Treat the underlying

cause. Urgent Na replacement is required if the patient is severely symptomatic and serum Na is less than 125 mmol/l. Seek expert guidance.

• If hyponatraemia is mild with no symptoms, and the patient is not dehydrated, treat by restricting fluid only. Start with 1 l/day, and reduce to 500 ml/day if there is no improvement within a few days.

• If the patient is dehydrated with normal renal function, give normal saline (0.9%).

Note: beware of correcting hyponatraemia too rapidly. This can cause central pontine myelinolysis with irreversible brain damage. IV hypertonic saline (5% saline at 70 mmol Na/hour) is rarely required unless the patient is fitting or unconscious. Discuss with your senior.

Hints

• Hyponatraemia due to ectopic ADH secretion may be the first sign of a small cell carcinoma of the lung (oat cell carcinoma).

• SIADH can only be diagnosed if the patient is hyponatraemic *and* the urine is more concentrated than the plasma.

• Mild hyponatraemia is frequently seen in severely ill patients ('sick cell' syndrome) but rarely requires treatment.

Transfusions

While blood transfusions are common in hospital, always be alert to transfusion reactions. Remember to reassure your patient that all blood is tested for HIV and other viral infections.

Blood transfusions

For chronic stable anaemia (see Anaemia p. 37)

1 Estimate the red cell deficit (1 unit of packed cells raises the Hb by 1 g/dl).
2 In general:
• Transfuse the patient to above 8 g/dl if they have a reversible cause of anaemia.
• Transfuse to above 10 g/dl if they have an irreversible cause of anaemia (e.g. myelodysplasia).
3 Check the patient's pulse, BP, JVP and chest for basal crackles as a baseline before transfusing.
4 The rate of transfusion will depend on the clinical setting and the presence or absence of heart disease.
• Transfuse slowly (each unit over 4–6 hours) in the elderly.
• Give frusemide 20–40 mg PO before the first unit and then with alternate bags if you are concerned about heart failure.
• If the patient becomes fluid overloaded, give frusemide 40 mg IV (do not mix in the bag). Repeat as necessary.
5 If the patient has had a previous transfusion reaction, give hydrocortisone (100 mg IV) and chlorpheniramine (10 mg IV) *before* the transfusion. This is often necessary in patients who have had multiple transfusions.

Hints

• Don't transfuse a new patient with chronic anaemia without checking iron and TIBC, B_{12} and folate (see Anaemia p. 37).
• Don't transfuse blood through lines

used for solutions containing dextrose, as this causes red cells to clump.

In the acute setting

1 Estimate how many units of blood the patient will need. In the acute setting, the Hb level lags the actual red cell loss by 12–24 hours.
2 Packed cells have few clotting factors and platelets. Therefore, for transfusions of more than 4 units, check the INR and APTT, and add 1–2 units of FFP for every 4 units of packed cells.
3 Transfuse to above 8 g/dl. Re-check the FBC daily.

Hints

• In acute and subacute bleeds, the MCV is normal.
• Remember hidden fractures in the elderly. The thigh can conceal 2 litres of blood.

Platelet transfusions

Indications

• Platelet count $<20 \times 10^9/l$, or $<40 \times 10^9/L$ and the patient is at risk of bleeding (e.g. going for major surgery).
• Thrombocytopenia or dysfunctional platelets with active bleeding.

Do

To order platelets, you need to know the patient's blood group but a cross-match is not necessary. If the patient has had a previous platelet transfusion reaction (common), administer hydrocortisone (100 mg IV) and chlorpheniramine (10 mg IV) before the transfusion. If the patient has had previous severe reactions, discuss HLA-matched platelets with the haematologist (they are very expensive).

Hint

• Platelet clumping often leads to erroneously low platelet counts. Always ask the haematologist to confirm an unexpectedly low count by manual differentiation.

Transfusion reactions

Slow rising fever <40 °C

A fever of up to 40 °C is very common during transfusions. It is treated by slowing the transfusion and giving paracetamol (1 g 4–6-hourly) if the patient is otherwise well.

Severe reaction

If the patient has a rapid T spike > 39 °C at the beginning of a transfusion, a T >40 °C at any time, an urticarial rash or wheezing and hypotension (anaphylaxis):
1 Stop the transfusion immediately. Send the bag and line to the lab for analysis.
2 Give the patient hydrocortisone 200 mg IV and chlorpheniramine 10 mg IV stat.
3 If the patient deteriorates or becomes hypotensive, call for immediate help and give 0.5–1.0 ml of a 1 : 1000 solution of adrenaline IM.
4 Monitor closely (risk of shock and acute renal failure).

Table 7.8 Differential diagnoses of oliguria/anuria.

Pre-renal	Renal	Post-renal
Hypovolaemia/hypotension • Occult bleed • Dehydration • Cardiac failure	*Nephrotoxic drugs* • Aminoglycosides • IV contrast dyes • Penicillins • Sulphonamides • NSAIDs	*Blocked catheter* *Retention* Prostate, tumour, idiopathic
Apparent intravascular hypovolaemia • 'Leaky capillaries' • Septicaemia • Pancreatitis • Post-major surgery • CCF, liver failure	*Systemic diseases* SLE, malignant hypertension etc. Interstitial nephritis	
Renal artery occlusion Emboli, aortic dissection		

Urine, low output (oliguria/anuria)

Oliguria is defined as a urine output of less than 500 ml in 24 hours. The minimum urine output is 0.5 ml/kg/hour (35 ml/hour in a 70 kg patient). Urgent assessment is required for an output of less than 20 ml/hour, a daily output of less than 500 ml, or for painful urinary retention (see Table 7.8).

On the ward

1 Check first for post-renal causes:
• Palpate the patient's abdomen for a distended bladder. Catheterize if the patient is in urinary retention. Remember to do a PR in men and PV in woman once the bladder is relieved, to exclude prostatic disease and pelvic masses respectively.
• If the patient is already catheterized, ask the nurse to do a small volume (100 ml) bladder wash-out to make sure that it isn't blocked.

2 Check for hypovolaemia and sepsis:
• Check BP, pulse, T and JVP.
• Assess fluid balance. Remember to include unrecorded losses (sweating, incontinence, etc.).
• Consider sepsis.
• If the patient is hypovolaemic, challenge with 500 ml IV normal saline over 30 minutes. If there is no urinary response, re-check their JVP and repeat the fluid challenge if it is low (and there is no risk of inducing CCF). In patients with poor cardiac function give 200 ml challenges. Consider a central line to monitor the CVP if the patient is acutely unwell.

3 Check for CCF:
• Oliguria indicates very poor cardiac output. Management should be discussed with your senior.

4 If you are unsure of the cause, get senior advice and do the following urgently:
• C&E and urea. A creatinine : urea

ratio of less than 10:1 (i.e. urea disproportionately raised) suggests a pre-renal cause.

• Urinary Na. A urinary Na of less than 15 mmol/l suggests pre-renal causes; more than 20 mmol/l suggests renal causes.

• Urine microscopy.

Hints

• Remember to alter the doses of renally excreted drugs if the patient has prolonged oliguria. Patients with peripheral oedema may still be hypovolaemic.

• Never use K-containing solutions for fluid challenges, as the impaired kidney may not be able to clear K.

• In a patient with oliguria or anuria (with a near-empty bladder), catheters can be very uncomfortable. This is relieved by a bladder washout. A washout will also exclude a blocked catheter as a cause for poor urine output.

Basic emergency routine

• If the patient is flat or very ill, get help fast and don't hesitate to call the crash team if you feel the patient is deteriorating. Check ABC.

• Briefly check for the 6 'H's: Hypoglycaemia, Hypotension, Hypovolaemia, Hypothermia, Hypoxia, and Arrhythmias (Heart). Check the BP (lying and sitting) and JVP, look for cyanosis and measure the respiratory rate. A good way to do the latter is to breathe with the patient. Do a blood glucose stick, ECG, pulse oximeter reading and consider doing a blood gas and rectal temperature. Check urine output.

• Ensure good IV access and consider a catheter and O_2. Monitor the patient's condition (quarter to half-hourly observations, ECG monitor, urine output) and do baseline investigations (see below).

• If the patient is well or stable you have time for a more thorough history and examination, although this does not mean a full CNS examination at 2 am (unless the problem is neurological!). For stable patients, urgent investigations are usually unnecessary and impede technicians' processing real emergencies. Before ordering new tests in the middle of the night, look at recent baseline tests and consider how new information will change management. If a test is not urgent but you don't want to forget it, write out the card for the morning and write in the notes.

Chapter 8: Death and dying

Approximately 65% of people die in hospital in the UK. Caring for dying people is stressful. Evidence suggests that medical students and junior doctors come to terms with mortality much younger than most people.

There are five elements to good terminal care: communication, pain control, symptom control, good prescribing knowledge and self care.

Communication

Breaking bad news

Breaking bad news is difficult but important. Contrary to popular opinion, people remember how bad news was related to them. While every situation demands a unique approach, the following may be helpful:

• If you are uncertain about how to start, talk to the patient's nurse. It is generally a good idea to ask nurses what they think the patient knows before seeing the patient. Take a nurse with you to the bedside.
• If possible, take the patient to a private room to tell them bad news.
• Have tissues handy.
• Try to hand your bleep to a nurse or colleague for at least 15–20 minutes.

• If you're unsure about how to proceed, it can be helpful to ask the patient 'What have you been told?'.
• Don't be afraid to give information. Studies show that people almost always want more information than doctors give them.[1]
• Watch and listen to the patient carefully for clues about how much information they want. If they indicate that they do not want to know everything at once, you may be more effective by feeding them information over several days.

> **Useful questions to assess how much someone wants to hear**
> 1 What have you been told?
> 2 Are you the sort of person who wants to know exactly what's going on?
> 3 Would you like me to tell you the full details of the diagnosis/results?
> 4 Do you want me to go on?

• Tell the truth and answer questions directly if asked (the patient may have been waiting all week to talk to you). Be ready to answer questions and to admit uncertainty. People are usually willing, even in the face of their own death, to cope with honest uncertainty. Have all investigations and findings to hand.
• Avoid using medical jargon.

[1]In 1961, 90% of doctors thought that patients were better off not being told about terminal disease, compared with 3% in 1979. Martin J. (1993) Lying to patients: can it ever be justified? *Nursing Standard* 7, 29–31.

• Write down relevant information and consider drawing diagrams to explain what you are saying more clearly (about 60% of spoken information is lost). Be prepared to repeat yourself many times.

• Ask the patient to write down questions they might have over the next few days. Give them your name or that of a colleague so that they can contact a doctor if they need to.

• Find out if the patient wants you to break the news to their relatives.

• Write in the notes what you have told the patient. This saves embarrassment for the team and sets a baseline for future explanations.

• Tell the nurses what you have told the patient. They can follow up with further information and support.

• Consider other people who can help with breaking bad news: other doctors, nurses, chaplain (about 25% of families accept chaplaincy support)[2], GP, nurse, police, social worker, support groups.

Ongoing communication with dying patients

• Pay a quick visit to the patient's bedside the next day (or at night if you're on call). Ask them how they're feeling and if they have any questions.

• Pain causes fear and anxiety, which may lead to the patient being withdrawn or aggressive. If you are not getting very far with a patient, remember to ask if they are in pain, or if they are frightened that they might develop severe pain. Reassure them that pain can be controlled; it is one of the most important con-

tributions you can make to a dying patient.

• If someone's English is poor, ask the nurses or switchboard to help you to find an interpreter. Most hospitals have a list of employees who can interpret for you.

• Be alert to attention-seeking symptoms, such as headaches and insomnia, which are probably better treated with TLC than pills. A direct approach is usually the best one. A colleague once had a patient who had 22 symptoms in 24 hours and wouldn't leave the nurses alone. The patient had been told that she had metastatic cancer that week. The doctor asked her outright 'How are you feeling about having secondaries?'. She burst into tears and told her she was terrified of dying—and stopped calling the nurses.

• Maintaining continuity of care, despite ward staff changes, is especially important for dying patients. Tell patients and relatives that you are going home for the weekend or on holiday, and the name of the doctor who will replace you.

• There are several stages of dying, including anger and denial. Pitch your information and communication to wherever the person is today. (This is easier said than done—remember to consider where you are at today too!)

• Do not be surprised by dying patients' aggressive or abnormal behaviour. This is when they need acceptance the most. Don't take it personally—and check that there is no physical cause (e.g. pain, hypoxia).

• Many dying people say that the most hurtful and distressing thing for them is avoidance and silence. Although it is of-

[2] Burgess K. (1992) Supporting bereaved relatives in A&E. *Nursing Standard* **6**, 36–39.

ten hard to do, allow patients to discuss dying with you (see below).
• Look patients in the eye when you talk to them.
• Reassure people that pain and other distressing symptoms can be treated.
• Check that the patient does not have awful images of dying patients from films!

Five questions to ask dying patients

1 What have they most enjoyed in their life? Ask them to describe it to you.

2 What would they like someone to hear, that they have never said?

3 What would they most like to say to people they love that they have never said? Ask them if there is any way they can communicate this (e.g. write a card, phone them from the ward, ask them to visit).

4 What are they most frightened of? You may be able to reassure them about pain and symptom control.

5 What do patients need to do (in practical terms) before they die? Talk to support staff (nurses, MacMillan nurses, social workers) and relatives about making this happen. It is very difficult for people to do things from a hospital bed.

Hint

Woolley and colleagues (1989) interviewed parents about their experiences of the way in which they were told of their children's life threatening illnesses. This article is well worth reading and pinning to your wall, as it gives an excellent, boxed outline of how to impart really difficult news. The reference is: Woolley H., Stein A., Forrest G.C., Baum J.D. (1989) Imparting the diagnosis of life threatening illness in children. *British Medical Journal* 298, 1632–1636.

Difficult situations

• Try turning difficult questions for you back to the patient. For example, you can ask them: 'What makes you ask that question?'[3]
• If family members make it clear to you that they don't want the patient to know that they are going to die, ask your senior or nurses for help. The relatives are not your primary responsibility, although obviously you have to work with them. You can point out that it is your duty to inform patients of their condition.
• Write down relatives' concerns in the patient's notes.

Mistakes we've made: avoid them!

• Don't under-estimate how much caring for dying patients can affect you. If you feel irritable or low, don't give yourself a hard time.
• Avoid medical jargon.
• Don't overwhelm patients and families with big doses of information at once. Try to give information in bite-size chunks.
• Consider writing things down and drawing clear diagrams for patients to look at after you've gone.
• Don't leave patients waiting. If you

[3]Macguire P., Faulkner A. (1988) Communicate with cancer patients: Handling bad news and difficult questions. *British Medical Journal* 297, 970–974.

promise to return, do so. People stay awake waiting for doctors to return.
• Never say 'Nothing can be done' or give the patient the impression that the medical staff have lost interest in them. Symptoms and distress can always be alleviated. Someone can always be present.
• Contrary to intuition, dying patients do not need to eat. It can be cruel to make them do so.
• Never give patients a 'date of death'. You will probably be wrong. Also, it is awful for all concerned if the patient lingers on after they 'should have died'.

Pain control (see Pain Control p. 126)

Pain is one of the things that dying patients are most afraid of. You can help them enormously, but you may need help:
• Use the pain clinic and ask for senior advice sooner rather than later if pain control is difficult.
• Remember the person may not admit to being in pain (check their pulse).
• Reassure patients that severe pain can be controlled, however severe.

Symptom control (listed alphabetically in Chapter 7)

The *BNF* has a fabulous, two page section on symptom control in terminal care (look under 'Terminal care' in the index) which we have not tried to replicate for fear of being too quickly outdated.

Prescribing for the dying

• Many drugs are available as suppositories, which are useful if the patient cannot swallow or is vomiting.
• Keep drugs as simple as possible. Discontinue when close to death.
• Keep analgesia continuous. IV or SC opiate infusions are useful for this as are PRN doses to back up regular doses of analgesia. Nurses will usually set up infusions for you. In dying patients, the ultimate aim is pain control and quality, not quantity of life. Discuss pain management with the nurses so that they don't simply stop infusions to avoid respiratory depression.
• Consider PCA. Discuss with the ward pharmacist.
• Consider withdrawing IV fluids but discuss with seniors and relatives first.
• Infusion pump troubleshooting:
  1 Light not flashing–pump not plugged in; battery inserted wrongly.
  2 Infusion running too fast or too slowly syringe incorrectly inserted, rate wrongly set, tubing kinked or blocked; needle site tissued.

Support for the dying and for you

Hospice (NHS or non-NHS); chaplain; hospital bereavement officer (if you have one).
CRUSE (widowed people caring for the newly bereaved), Cruse House, 126 Sheen Road, Richmond, Surrey TW9 1UR, Tel: 0181-940 4818.
MacMillan Nurses (nurses specially trained for palliative care), part of

MacMillan Cancer Relief, Anchor House, 15–19 Britten Street, London SW3 3TZ, Tel: 0171-351 7811.

Marie Curie Cancer Care, Marie Curie Memorial Foundation, Head Office, 28 Belgrave Square, London SW1X 8QG, Tel: 0171-235 3325.

Some questions to ask yourself if *you* feel excessively miserable caring for dying patients
• Make a list of five 'significant losses' you have experienced. Write down positive outcomes that arose from those situations, and identify ways in which you developed as a result.
• Do the same exercise for 'necessary losses' – those which you had no control over.[4]

DEATH

If the patient dies, don't panic. While really sad, death is often merciful when people have been suffering – for them, their relatives and ward staff. You can make a big difference to relatives if you handle the paperwork efficiently, allowing them to proceed with the funeral.

[4]Hasler K. (1994) Bereavement counselling. Continuing Education article series (article 306). *Nursing Standard* 7, 31–35.

What to do when a patient dies

1 See the body.

2 Confirm death: fixed and dilated pupils, no respiratory effort for 3 minutes, no pulse, no heart sounds for 1 minute.
• If you are unsure, do an ECG or look at the fundi. The blood in the retinal veins separates into discrete blotches after death.

3 Write in the notes: 'Called to confirm death. No vital signs.'

4 Sign your name clearly with your bleep number. It is important that coroners and bereavement officers can contact you if necessary.

5 Note date and time of confirmation of death.

6 If possible write down the cause(s) of death.

7 NOTE WHETHER OR NOT THE PATIENT IS FITTED WITH A PACEMAKER OR RADIOACTIVE IMPLANT. If the patient is to be cremated, pacemakers and radioactive implants *must* be removed or they blow up in the incinerator at considerable cost to yourself. It is easiest to check for these while you still have the patient and the notes in front of you. If you do not check this now you will have to chase the body and the notes in the morgue in order to sign the cremation form.

8 Liaise with nurses about calling next of kin. Nurses usually tell the next of kin and meet them on the ward, but relatives may want to see you.

9 Note the GP's telephone number and name. You should call him or her at the earliest opportunity to let them know so they don't make a faux pas

when they next see the relatives ('So how's so and so doing in hospital?').

10 Write 'GP informed' in notes.

11 Ask your senior early whether or not a PM is desirable, and what cause(s) of death should be written on the death certificate.

Telling relatives about the patient's death

1 Wherever possible, inform the relatives that their loved one is close to death. Ask relatives whether they want to be contacted in the middle of the night, establish the next of kin and how they can be contacted.

2 After death, ask the nurses whether they have told the relatives about the patient's death. They will often do so— sometimes before you make it to the ward.

3 If it is up to you to inform relatives, make sure you contact the patient's designated 'next of kin'. Ask the nurses who this is, or look in the nursing or medical notes.

4 It is usually best to tell the next of kin what has happened over the phone (rather than just asking them to come in urgently). Sometimes people don't want to see the body or would rather wait until morning.

5 If you receive the relatives, take them to a private room. If they have come a long way they might be grateful for a cup of tea.

6 Try to establish:
- If the body is to be cremated or buried. If the former, you will need to fill out a cremation form (see below).
- If the relatives will consent to a post mortem (see below).

Post mortems

- Preferably before the patient dies, ask your colleagues if they want a PM so that you can ask the relatives when the patient dies.
- PMs requested by the coroner are mandatory by law. Otherwise, you cannot force a next of kin to agree to a PM. Many people will oblige if you explain why you want one, particularly if it is a limited PM.
- Send case notes (complete with recent investigation results), the next of kin's consent form and a brief synopsis of the patient's history and hospital progress to the PM room, together with your name and bleep number.
- Request that the pathologist bleeps you or your senior with the results.

Death certificates

Only doctors who have seen the patient within 14 days before death are legally allowed to sign a death certificate. The next of kin must take this to the Registrar of Births and Deaths within 5 days (8 days in Scotland) in a sealed envelope. Give the signed death certificate to either the nurses, the ward clerk or the family.

- If there is no next of kin, you must ensure that the death certificate is sent to the registrar.

Writing the death certificate

Make sure you fill in the death certificate correctly or you may be recalled by the registrar and delay the funeral. (Don't be too hard on yourself if you do make mistakes, as it is not the simplest document to fill out.)

1 Part one: Fill in the sequence of conditions that caused the patient's death. *1a)* is the condition that caused death. Causes of death are recognized pathological states, such as MI. The cause of death must not be too general. For example, organ failure is not an acceptable cause. Other unacceptable causes are tabulated below. Ask your senior or ring the registrar if you are unsure about how to describe the cause of death.

Unacceptable 'causes' of death	
Asphyxia	Hepatic failure
Asthenia	Hepatorenal failure
Brain failure	Kidney failure
Cachexia	Renal failure
Cardiac arrest	Respiratory arrest
Cardiac failure	Shock
Coma	Syncope
Debility	Uraemia
Exhaustion	Vagal inhibition
Heart failure	Vaso-vagal attack

1b) and c) are diseases underlying this condition. For example, if the cause of death was MI, the underlying disease might be ischaemic heart disease, or chronic hypertension.

2 Part two: Fill in other diseases which were not directly linked with the cause of death in 1a), but which may have contributed to the patient's overall demise.

3 Sign the death certificate on the relevant part of the form.

4 Print your name, hospital and most recent medical qualification on the relevant part of the form.

5 Print the name of the patient's consultant on the relevant part of the form.

6 Fill in the counterfoil ('cheque-butt') part of death certificate. This retains the basic details of the death when the relatives have taken the main certificate.

7 Fill in the 'note to informant'. This is given to the next of kin.

• If you are unsure about any part of the death certificate, call the registrar's officer or talk to a colleague or bereavement officer. The registrar's office is in the phone book under 'Registrar of Births and Deaths'.

• Don't use abbreviations on the death certificate.

• If your hospital has a bereavement officer, he or she will usually discuss the request for a PM with the relatives and will help you with the death certificate.

• It is courteous to relatives to write the cause of death in lay-language (e.g. 'stroke' as well as cerebral infarction).

• If your patient was a war pensioner or serviceman/woman, you can influence whether or not their spouse continues to receive war widow(er)'s pension by what you write on the death certificate. This is especially important if the person died from war-related causes.

• Doctors must record diseases which may have been due to previous employment.

Referring to the coroner (Scotland: procurator fiscal)

1 To contact your local coroner or procurator, ask your senior, switchboard, the police station or directory enquiries for the phone number.

2 It is the statutory obligation of the Registrar of Births and Deaths, not you, to report suspect deaths to the coroner or procurator fiscal. However, it saves

time if you know what these are and can send the death certificate directly to the coroner. They are:
- Unknown cause of death.
- The patient was not seen by certifying doctor within 14 days of death.
- Death was caused by medical treatment (e.g. dying in theatre, or within 24 hours of an anaesthetic).
- Death was suspicious in any way.
- Death occurred within 24 hours of admission to hospital without a firm diagnosis being made.
- Death was caused by a road traffic accident, an industrial disease or accident, a domestic accident, violence, neglect, abortion, suicide or poisoning (including acute alcohol ingestion).
- Death occurred during legal custody.
- Where there is any claim for negligence against medical or nursing staff.
- Death may have occurred from industrial injury or employment.
- Death of a foster child, patient under Mental Health Act (1983), mental defectives, Service Pensioners.
3 The coroner can request:
- The issue of a normal death certificate.
- A PM.
- An inquest.
House Officers rarely have to deal with this. If in doubt, phone the coroner and discuss the case.

Cremation forms and fees

You receive approximately £36 for every cremation form you fill out. 'Crem forms' are legal documents to establish

beyond any doubt the deceased's identity, as incinerated bodies cannot be exhumed. If you have not seen the patient since death, you must pay a quick visit to the cold room so that you know you are signing the form for the right person.

Crem forms are straightforward to fill out, provided you are certain there are no radioactive or pacemaker implants in the body.
- Ensure you fill in the same cause(s) of death on the crem form that you did on the death certificate or you will be chased by the coroner.
- If in doubt, call the coroner's office or ask a medical colleague.
- If the family is poor you can forgo the crem fee. In some hospitals this is standard policy. If you choose not to accept crem fees, you need a tax exemption form from the morgue director or bereavement officer so that you don't get taxed for fees you haven't taken.
- Keep details of cremation fees you have taken as you need to declare them in your tax forms. Increasingly the Inland Revenue is checking up on doctors for non-declaration (see p. 202).

To check for pacemakers

- Feel the chest.
- Look through the notes for history of implantation of pacemaker or radioactive implant.
- Look for ECGs that will demonstrate an active pacemaker by small, regular vertical lines throughout the trace.
- The only sure-fire way to exclude a pacemaker is to see a recent chest X-ray. Make sure you see it before the radiology department removes it from the in-patient file.

Did you know:
- 600 000 people die in the UK each year.
- At least 1 500 000 people suffer major bereavement each year.
- There are 3 200 000 widows and 750 000 widowers: one woman in seven is a widow, one man in 28 is a widower.
- 180 000 children under 16 have lost a parent (Office of Population Censuses & Surveys and from DSS Statistics Office, Newcastle-Upon Tyne).

Further reading

There are many excellent books and articles on death and dying. Ask your librarian. Here are some useful articles for starters:

Buckman R. (1992) *How to Break Bad News. A Guide for Health Care Professionals*. Papermac, London.

Continuing Education article series on bereavement counselling. (1994) *Nursing Standard*.

Cooke M., Cooke H., Glucksman E. (1992) Management of sudden bereavement in the accident and emergency department. *British Medical Journal* **304**, 1207–1209.

Egan G. (1990) *The Skilled Helper. A Systematic Approach to Effective Helping*. 4th edn. Brookes-Cole, Pacific Grove CA.

Macguire P., Faulkner L. (1988) Communicate with cancer patients: handling bad news and difficult patients. *British Medical Journal* **297**, 907–909.

McLauchlan C. (1990) Handling distressed relatives and breaking bad news. *British Medical Journal* **301**, 1145–1149.

Raphael B. (1984) *The Anatomy of Bereavement*. Hutchinson, London.

Thayre K., Hadfield-Law L. (1993) Never going to be easy: Giving bad news. RCN Nursing Update; Continuing Education article series *Nursing Standard* **8**, 3–13.

Worden W. (1991) *Grief Counselling and Grief Therapy. A Handbook for the Mental Health Practitioner*. 2nd edn. Springer, London.

Chapter 9: Drugs

Don't worry if pharmacology seems a long time ago. Prescribing and giving drugs is not difficult.

General

• The most useful pharmacology tip is: *always refer to the BNF if in any doubt about any drug*. As an House Officer, you will rarely be expected to prescribe drugs that are not in the *BNF*. Also, read the *BNF* for entertainment during long ward rounds; it contains lots of useful information. For example, it contains prescribing guidelines for the elderly, the terminally ill and children.

• Make the most of your ward pharmacist. Not only are pharmacists happy to discuss patient management and find alternatives for problematic drugs (or patients!) but they are often willing to find recent articles and other information about specific drugs for you. This can be very useful for clarifying unusual side effects and for academic talks!

• For easy reference, make yourself a chart of common drugs and doses used on the wards, and stick it on the front of your folder or filofax. It is particularly useful to do this for infusion dosages, which can be painstaking to look up every time you make up an infusion. We have refrained from providing such lists in this book because every hospital's protocol is different and drug doses vary over time. As always, check the *BNF*!

Prescribing drugs

Drug charts

Drug charts are straightforward to fill out. Basically, there are three parts to a drug chart:

1 A place for regular drugs.
2 A place for 'PRN' or 'when required' drugs.
3 A place for one-off drugs.

For each section of the chart, you need to fill in the date, the generic name of each drug, its dose, how frequently it should be prescribed, and your signature. Abbreviations for prescribing are shown in Table 9.1.

Tips for filling in drug charts

• Write legibly. Other people have to administer drugs that you prescribe.

• In particular, take care in writing dose amounts and units. Micrograms (abbreviated mcg) can easily be mistaken for milligrams (mg); the *BNF* advises that 'micrograms' and 'units' be written in full. (A doctor was sued when a patient was given 125 mg of digoxin by a nurse who misread the scrawled 'mcg'. She had to open many packets of the drug to give such a dose, so also ended up in the dock for failure of common sense.)

• Develop a good relationship with the ward pharmacist. S/he reviews all drug charts and will bleep you if you

Table 9.1 Abbreviations for prescribing drugs.

Abbreviation	Meaning
ac (ante cibum)	before food
pc (post cibum)	after food
bd (bis die)	take twice daily
mane	take in the morning
nocte	take in the evening
od	take once daily
prn (pro re nata)	take when required
qds	take four times a day
stat	take straight away
tds	take three times a day
ī īī īīī	one tablet two tablets three tablets
x/7, y/52, z/12	x days, y weeks, z months

prescribe anything idiotic. Similarly, nurses, who administer many drugs, will usually let you know if you have made a prescription error.

• Hospital pharmacists usually use green ink. To avoid confusion, use a different colour when writing on drug charts.

• If drug administration is complicated, write additional instructions on the drug chart. There is no harm in writing extra notes to nurses and doctors on the drug chart. In fact it is legally advisable to do so.

Writing prescriptions

Pre-registration House Officers are only permitted to write prescriptions for the hospital pharmacy. However if you do need to write a prescription on plain paper the essential ingredients are:
• Date.
• Name of patient.
• Address of patient.
• Generic drug name and amount.
• Dose/day.
• Your signature.
For example:

> 27/8/96
> Mr JS
> 17 SWP Road
> Oxford OX1
> Carbimazole 10 mg bd
> (Your signature and printed name)

Controlled drugs

Prescriptions for take-home controlled drugs have to be written in a particular way, otherwise the pharmacy will send the prescription back. This wastes a spectacular amount of time. To write a controlled drug prescription:
• The prescription must be in your handwriting – don't use sticky labels.
• Include:
  • Date.
  • Name of patient.
  • Address of patient.
  • Generic drug name and amount (e.g. '10 mg').
  • Dose/day
  • Number of tablets in **both** numbers and letters (e.g. '10/ten tablets').
  • Your signature and printed name.
For example:

5/4/96
Mr TSD
2 Tatelman Street
Wolfchester WC5

MST continuous tablets 10 mg
10/ten tablets
10 mg twice daily for 5 days

(Your signature and printed name)

Verbals

In many hospitals you can prescribe drugs for patients 'verbally' over the phone to nurses. Typical verbal requests might be 'Mr Smith has a headache. Could he have two paracetamol please?' The nurse writes your prescription in the drug chart, with a small note saying 'Dr X will sign this'. Verbals are great for relatively harmless drugs, such as one-off doses of paracetamol or aspirin, or for doses of necessary drugs when you have been held up and coming to the ward is monumentally inconvenient.
• Check hospital policy. Increasingly verbals are not allowed by Trusts.
• It is important to sign verbal requests on the drug chart as soon as possible. Should any problems arise in the interim, the nurse who took the verbal is liable for damages. Because of this, some nurses refuse to take verbals and insist you come to the ward to sign the drug before it is given.
• Nurses will usually refuse to accept verbals if they think the patient should be seen by a doctor before taking the drug. While this can be frustrating, remember that nurses' scruples provide a big safety net for you. Everyone remembers times when they were glad that nurses forced them to question what they were doing.

Giving drugs

Nurses give oral drugs, suppositories, SC and IM drugs. In some hospitals nurses also give IV drugs. Usually the House Officer makes up infusions and may give IV drugs.
• Use a metal file to open difficult glass drug vials by scratching the neck with the file, and snapping it off. Nurses usually have a file stashed somewhere on the ward.
• Wear gloves or use your non-dominant hand when opening multiple vials. Your dominant hand's index finger can get very chaffed with minute glass splinters if you snap open many glass vials consecutively.
• Avoid using normal saline as a dilutant for drugs in patients with liver failure; 5% dextrose is usually adequate.
• Avoid dextrose in patients with diabetic coma! Give normal saline instead. Refer to the *BNF* for alternative dilutants for different drugs.

Drug infusions

Continuous infusions are easy to make up, but they are a complete pain at 4 am. Always make up midnight infusions before going to bed. This is particularly true of morphine, dopamine and GTN infusions, which you will be called out of bed for otherwise.

To make up an infusion

1 Find the vial of drug in the drug cupboard. Check the dosage and the expiry date.
2 Open the vial (use a file if difficult – see above).

3 Draw up the drug into a suitably large syringe, usually 50 ml.

4 Draw into the syringe the required amount of dilutant fluid. Usually normal saline, water for injections or 5% dextrose, drawn from unopened (sterile) containers.

5 Label the syringe with a large sticky. Specify on the sticky:

• Date and time you made infusion up.

• Name of patient.

• Amount of drug in amount of dilutant (e.g. 50 mg GTN in 50 ml normal saline).

• Rate at which solution should run (e.g. 2 ml/hour).

• Your signature.

6 If the infusion is not needed for a few hours, put it in the fridge and let the nurses know where it is.

Prescribing drug infusions

1 Prescribe infusions on the fluid section of the drug chart. In some hospitals this is a separate sheet at the end of the patient's bed.

2 Write: a units of b drug in x ml of y dilutant to run at z ml/hour.

e.g. 25 000 units of heparin in 50 ml N/saline. Run at 2 ml/hour.

3 To avoid confusion, convert the amount of drug/hour to the amount of infusion to be given every hour (i.e. ml/hour, not mg/hour). To do this, ask yourself the following questions:

• How many units of drug should the patient get per hour?

e.g. 1000 units heparin/hour

• How many units of drug are there per ml of infusion?

e.g. 25 000 units/50 ml infusion = 500 units/ml

• Therefore, how many ml do I need to give so that the patient gets the right amount of units per hour?

e.g. 1 000 units/hour ÷ 500 units/ml = 2 ml/hour

4 You can always write additional instructions on the drug chart regarding infusion administration.

e.g. 50 mg GTN in 50 ml N/saline; run at 1–10 ml/hour titrated against chest pain.

Administering infusions

If the nurses are willing to administer infusions, all you have to do is let them know that you have made up the infusion, and where they can find it.

• Otherwise, get a nurse to show you how to set up a pump (e.g. Vickers). It is not difficult. Basically you insert the syringe into the pump with the drug label facing outwards, set the rate on the machine, plug it in and turn it on. You also have to remember to connect the patient to the syringe!

• Infusions can run through central or peripheral lines. Many infusions can run concurrently with other drugs through three-way taps or multiple-tap ('traffic light') giving sets. These are simple to set up with initial nurse supervision.

• Some infusions cannot be mixed with others. The most problematic are those containing collating ions, such as Ca. Unfortunately these require a second Venflon or need flushing with heparanized saline (Hepsal) or saline before another drug is administered through the same line.

• Place the syringe driver below the level of the patient's head to avoid the risk of siphoning.

Intravenous drugs

If you are in a hospital where nurses do not administer IV drugs then you need to mix them with dilutant and give them yourself. This means doing an IV drug round 3 to 4 times daily.

1 Ensure the patient really needs the drug IV. Most drugs may be given PO, PR, SC or IM. It is time consuming for you and expensive for the NHS to give drugs IV.

2 Read the instructions in the drug packet. Some drugs can be injected directly into the patient's vein. However, they usually need to be diluted first.

Liquid drugs not requiring dilution

If the drug can be given without dilution, draw it up with a small syringe and inject it over the recommended time. Some drugs must be given slowly to avoid anaphylaxis or pain in the patient's arm which they won't thank you for. Most drugs can be given quite quickly (over less than 30 seconds–1 minute). Read the *BNF* and the drug's instructions.

Liquid drugs requiring dilution

If the drug comes in liquid form which needs diluting, this is easily done by drawing the drug into a suitably large syringe (e.g. 10 or 20 ml), and then drawing in sterile saline or water for injection (available in small, sterile vials in the drug cupboard).

• Always use sterile fluid when diluting drugs; patients can get septic from once-sterile fluid that has been lying around unsealed.

Powdered drugs

If the drug comes in a vacuum container as a powder, you need to dissolve it with a solute, such as water for injection. Most antibiotics come this way. To avoid giving yourself and the ward a drug shower (Fig. 9.1):

1 Draw the required amount of water for injection into a suitably large syringe through a needle. Tap or push the end of the syringe to expel any air, so that the water is flush with the top of the syringe.

2 Remove the flip-off plastic top of the drug vial.

3 Push the needle through the rubber top of the drug vial and withdraw some air to create a vacuum inside the vial.

4 Tap or tilt the syringe so that the withdrawn air moves through the water to the back of the syringe.

5 Inject the water into the vial, with the assistance of the vacuum you have just created. You may need to repeat this several times.

6 When you have injected enough water, shake the vial (or leave it to dissolve while you do something else).

7 Withdraw the needle. Draw some air into the syringe. Re-introduce the needle into the vial through the rubber top and inject some air to create positive pressure inside the vial.

8 Turn the vial upside down and withdraw the dissolved drug from the vial with the assistance of the positive pressure.

9 Don't worry if on first attempts you spray yourself, the desk and unwary passers-by with the drug. You will soon be able to do the whole thing perfectly in your sleep.

Fig. 9.1 Preparing powdered drugs.

Specific drug topics

Antibiotics

• Check your hospital drug guidelines with seniors and pharmacologists. Each hospital has particular protocols which are usually published.

• Always ask patients if they have known antibiotic (penicillin) allergy before prescribing penicillin or cephalosporin antibiotics. Erythromycin is a reasonable alternative to ampicillin and related drugs. Also be alert to pseudomembranous colitis (send stool specimen for *Clostridium difficile*) if the patient develops diarrhoea and fever.

• Common antibiotic side effects include diarrhoea and vaginal (and other) candidiasis (thrush). Consider prescribing an anticandidiasis pessary/cream on the PRN side of the drug chart.
• Warn women taking the oral contraceptive pill that antibiotics (and other drugs affecting liver metabolism) reduce its efficacy.
• Consider giving at least 24 hours IV treatment if the patient is very unwell.
• Check the *BNF* and local guidelines for the most current treatment of different infections.
• Gentamicin, netilmycin and vancomycin need regular peak and trough levels (see the *BNF* or phone pharmacology).

Standard treatments for common infections include
Chest infection
Oral amoxycillin (erythromycin if penicillin allergic)
Second choice: erythromycin or ciprofloxacin
You do not need to give erythromycin *and* amoxycillin unless there is consolidation

Severe infection or hospital acquired infection
IV cephalosporin, e.g. cefuroxime

Aspiration pneumonia
Amoxycillin and metronidazole

UTI
Oral trimethoprim *or* cephalosporin *or* ciprofloxacin

Cellulitis
Flucloxacillin and amoxycillin

Septicaemia
IV cefuroxime and gentamicin (see hospital policy)

Anticoagulation

House Officers are often required to anticoagulate patients following heart attacks, DVTs and PEs. Ask your colleagues for local protocols. These generally involve giving heparin and warfarin together, then stopping the heparin once the INR is high enough (i.e. when the warfarin begins to work).
1 Check that the patient has no bleeding disorder. Do FBC, INR and APTT.
2 Start the patient on a heparin pump (usually 25 000 units in 50 ml of normal saline, run at 2.8 ml/hour (1400 units/hour). Check the APTT at least once a day and adjust the heparin according to a sliding scale (see the *BNF*). Ideally, the APTT should hover around 1.5–2.5. The heparin should be stopped if the APTT is more than 7.
3 Start the patient simultaneously on warfarin. The standard protocol is:
• Give 10 mg of warfarin on the first day, 5 mg on the second and third, then adjust according to the INR. This protocol may need to be modified for the elderly, frail, those with liver disease and on liver-stimulating drugs. Check with your senior.
• You need to check the INR daily from the first dose. Reduce the warfarin dose if the INR rises too quickly or too high (e.g. above 5).
• The INR needs to be checked:
  Every day for 1 week
  Every week for 3 weeks
  Every month for 3 months
  Every 8 weeks after that
Always inform the GP in the dis-

charge summary that the patient has been started on warfarin and that the INR will need to be checked.

• You are usually aiming for an INR of 2–3 (but this varies depending on the condition; check the *BNF*).

• Clearly explain the potential side effects of warfarin to the patient and that they must inform their GP and any other health professional that they are taking warfarin. It is also advisable to tell the patient to keep tablets well hidden from small children.

• If the INR or APTT are too high, simply stop the warfarin and/or heparin. If the INR is greater than 10, or the patient is bleeding, give 4 units of FFP and recheck the clotting. A small dose (1–2 mg) of vitamin K will reverse the clotting in a few hours. Beware of giving higher doses as this prevents further anticoagulation for weeks. Always consult with a haematologist and colleagues if a patient is in danger of bleeding. Beware of anaphylaxis (be prepared to treat with O_2 and adrenaline, see p. 71). FFP can also be given stat to decrease a bleeding tendency. Heparin can be reversed with protamine sulphate. Use 1 mg protamine sulphate/100 iu of heparin, to a maximum of 50 mg. This should work within half an hour.

Anti-emetics (see Nausea and vomiting p. 71)

Digoxin

Digoxin is a commonly used drug to slow down the ventricular rate in atrial fibrillation. It is potentially dangerous with many side effects, such as fatigue, confusion. N&V, anorexia, diarrhoea and arrhythmias. Digoxin also interacts with many drugs (see the *BNF*). In particular, beware of drugs which lower K (e.g. diuretics), as hypokalaemia predisposes to digoxin toxicity.

How to digitalize (discuss with your senior first)

1 In the non-acute situation:

• Give the patient 125–250 µg (micrograms) of digoxin twice daily for 1 week. No loading dose is required.

• Reduce dose to once daily for maintenance. Digoxin maintenance dosage varies according to age, weight and renal function. In general:
Normal dose 125–375 µg.
In the elderly 62.5–125 µg.
If renal impairment, discuss with pharmacologist.

• If the patient experiences side effects, measure digoxin levels for toxicity. Digoxin-specific antibodies are now available as an antidote to digoxin poisoning.

2 In the acute situation (for more rapid control of the ventricular rate):

• Give 500 µg of digoxin 8-hourly until the rate is controlled (usually takes 3–4 doses), then give the maintenance dose (see above), or

• Give 500 µg IV and 500 µg orally at the same time, then continue with maintenance doses. This method is faster.

Night sedation (see Insomnia p. 68)

Be wary of giving night sedation without making sure that the patient does not need further medical attention or better day management.

Table 9.2 Therapeutic drug levels and sampling times.

Drug	Sampling time	Therapeutic range
Amiodarone	Any time when blood levels are stable (after 1 month)	0.6–2.5 mg/l
Carbamazepine	Peak 3 hours after dose	Single therapy: 8–12 mg/l Multiple therapy: 4–8 mg/l
Digoxin	At least 6 h after dose Check C&E and Ca, as toxicity is potentiated if Ca is high or K is low	0.8–2 µg/l
Gentamicin and tobramicin	Peak 1 hour after dose Trough (just before new dose)	Peak 5–10 mg/l Trough <2 mg/l
Lithium	12 hours after dose	0.4–1.0 mmol/l
Phenytoin	IV peak 2–4 hours after dose Oral peak 3–9 hours after dose	10–20 mg/l
Sodium valproate	Plasma levels are not a good guide to efficacy	
Vancomycin	Peak 1 hour after dose Trough Also check C&E for renal toxicity	25–40 mg/l 1 3 mg/l

Therapeutic drug levels

House Officers are sometimes required to check the blood levels of several commonly used drugs (Table 9.2). This involves liaising with the nurse giving the drug so that you can take blood for levels at the appropriate times (e.g. at peak and trough dosage times). Ask the biochemistry technicians which tube to use (usually a biochemistry tube).

Steroids (see The steroid patient p. 110)

Miscellaneous tips

• Metronidazole can be given easily and cheaply as a suppository. This is particularly useful after an appendicectomy, if the patient does not need a drip.
• Metronidazole bags for IV use can be requested from pharmacy. You can ask the pharmacist to add cefuroxime so that you don't have to do IV drug rounds for either (the nurses put them up). Store the bags in the fridge and watch the use-by date.
• If a drug risks causing anaphylaxis (e.g. phytomenadione), ensure that you

have adrenaline ready and a resuscitation trolley available. *Do not leave the ward for about 5 minutes after giving these drugs.*

• Any drug which is protein-based can cause anaphylaxis.

• Always consider prescribing laxatives prophylactically with opiate analgesia.

• Steroid conversion (also see p. 110): 0.75 mg dexamethasone = 5 mg prednisolone = 20 mg hydrocortisone = 25 mg cortisone.

• Consider pre-emptive prescribing (i.e. prescribing certain drugs on the PRN side of the chart for all patients without contraindications) to prevent nurses bleeping you and your colleagues: paracetamol, temazepam (see above), laxatives.

Chapter 10: Handle with care

Some patients require special attention as they are especially vulnerable due to physical or mental frailty, and stigma.

Alcoholism

Many more of your patients will be addicted to alcohol than you realize. To assess alcoholism, do the CAGE questionnaire[1], which is remarkably reliable for picking up alcoholism:

1 Have you ever felt you should C UT down on drinking?

2 Have people made you A NGRY by asking about your alcohol intake?

3 Have you ever felt G UILTY about your drinking?

4 Do you ever drink first thing in the morning (or take an E YE OPENER)?

Answering 'yes' to two or more of the above questions gives the patient an 80% chance of having an alcohol problem.

• Ask the patient for a typical day, with the amount and type of alcohol taken at each time.

• Tactfully ask relatives or friends about the patient if you suspect denial of alcoholism.

• Do an MCV (with FBC) and GGT. Both rise with prolonged use of alcohol, and take approximately 2–3 months to

[1] Mayfield D., McLeod G., Hall P. (1974) *American Journal of Psychiatry* **131**, 1121–1123.

return to normal following abstention. If these are raised, discuss the findings with the patient and your colleagues regarding further treatment.

• Women should not drink more than 14 units/week; men 21 units/week. One unit contains 8 g of alcohol. Drinks containing 1 unit of alcohol include a half pint of beer, a small glass of red or white wine, a single bar serving of spirits or sherry or fortified wine.

• Consider a nutritional screen and vitamin supplements (especially the B, D and K groups).

Alcohol withdrawal

Some patients will be admitted specifically to withdraw from alcohol; others will have their alcoholism unmasked in hospital. Always consider alcohol (and nicotine) withdrawal if your patient suddenly becomes unexpectedly ill or agitated.

• Ask your senior for local protocols.

• Watch for hypotension, dehydration, hypoglycaemia and electrolyte imbalance. Ensure 4 hourly observation and regular C&E, glucose, FBC.

• Prescribe chlormethiazole as shown in Table 10.1. Do not treat with chlormethiazole for more than 9 days. *Note that lorazepam is rapidly superceding the use of chlormethiazole in some centres. It is cheaper and more effective. Ask your senior for their preference.*

• Consider IV chlormethiazole if the patient is vomiting. A 0.8% infusion

Table 10.1 Prescribing chlormethiazole. Do not treat with chlormethiazole for more than 9 days.

Day	Number of chlormethiazole tablets	Tablet timing
Day 1	2–4	6 hourly
Day 2	2–3	6 hourly
Day 3	1–2	9 hourly
Days 4–9	Gradually decrease dose	

of chlormethiazole at 3–7.5 ml (24–60 mg)/minute, reducing to 0.5–1 ml (4–8 mg)/minute, should keep the patient lightly sedated. Consult with your senior before administering IV chlormethiazole. A resuscitation trolley must be available and frequent observations performed, as the patient may become too deeply sedated.

• Be careful with chlormethiazole. Patients should not drive for 48 hours after taking the last dose. Sedation may mask hepatic coma. Avoid prolonged use and abrupt withdrawal. Dependence becomes a problem after about 9 days.

• Randomized controlled trials suggest that patients are likely to do better if they are initially detoxified in hospital, as opposed to being managed solely in the community.[2]

Children

You may work with children as a surgical House Officer, although you are not expected to provide full paediatric care. These tips may help:

• Remove your white coat before working with children. It helps to avoid doctor phobia and unnecessary formality.

• For children under 14, get consent from parents/guardians while they are on the ward, or you will have to call them in from home.

• Minors between 14 and 16 can legally sign for themselves, but it is usually a good idea to get parental or guardian consent.

• Ask the anaesthetist to insert cannulae when the child is asleep for theatre, to minimize needle trauma and phobia.

• Use paediatric blood bottles (available on paediatric wards and in the paediatric room in casualty) to minimize blood letting.

• Use local anaesthetic cream before inserting cannulae and taking blood.

• Be cautious when prescribing IV fluids and drugs – different sized children have very different fluid and drug needs. Consult the *BNF* and colleagues if in doubt.

• If you are desperate for a vein, children under about 10 months have good scalp veins which can be accessed using a blue butterfly.

[2] Walsh D.C., *et al.* (1991) A randomized trial of treatment options for alcohol-abusing workers. *New England Journal of Medicine* **325**, 775–782.

Depression

People in hospital are often depressed–with good reason. Hospitals can be scary, lonely places even if you are well, let alone facing serious illness and death.

• Be alert to sudden mood changes and negative conversation. Ask patients about their fears. You may be able to help immediately with reassurance or liaisons with social workers, nurses, psychiatrists and medical colleagues.

• Interestingly, many elderly patients suffering from acute conditions such as MI or strokes have been recently bereaved. Your patient may be grieving.

• If your patient seems low, they may be suffering from occult pain, hypoxia, alcohol or drug withdrawal, electrolyte and thyroid imbalances, as well as concerns about employment, home care and other likely worries.

• Alert psychiatrists and colleagues if you think a patient is in danger of attempting suicide (see pp. 19–20).

Elderly patients

Like children, elderly patients can present with non-specific, under-stated symptoms. Elderly patients are often stoical and may hide quite severe pain.

1 Monitor vital signs. Breathe with the patient to exclude quiet tachypnoea. Consider checking rectal temperature.

2 Go through a checklist of systems to make sure you're not missing something serious. In particular, watch for:

• Fractures: old people often don't complain of pain. *Look* at the limbs (especially the hips, legs and wrists) and feel for crepitus.

• Hypoxia: people may present with euphoria. Measure the respiratory rate and do pulse oximetry or blood gases if concerned.

• Fluid overload and electrolyte imbalance: check IV fluids, electrolytes and slow down or stop fluids if necessary. A basic IV fluid regime for elderly people is:

Normal saline
    500 ml + KCl 20 mM
        Over 6 hours
Normal saline
    500 ml + KCl 20 mM
        Over 6 hours
5% Dextrose 500 ml + KCl 20 mM
        Over 6 hours
5% Dextrose 500 ml
        Over 6 hours

and monitor electrolytes daily. Reconsider whether the patient needs IV fluids.

• Hypothermia: consider checking rectal temperature.

• Malnutrition: look for flaky skin, poor gums, unhealed bruises or scratches. Consider a nutritional screen.

• K-wasting with diuretics. Check K and supplement orally if necessary. Be careful not to produce hyperkalaemia. If you send the patient home with K supplements, be sure to notify both the patient and the GP, so K can be monitored.

• Infantilization of elderly patients. Remember that 80% of elderly patients live at home. Only 14% of people over 75 have any form of dementia. Be careful not to treat elderly people like children.

Haemophiliacs

All in all, haemophiliacs get a bad deal. The majority of adult UK haemophiliacs are Hep B/C and/or HIV-positive. Bad haemophilia can be crippling, as members of various royal families can testify. This is one group to communicate openly with, and take the following precautions.

Taking blood

• Minimize taking blood. Question your colleagues if they have requested frequent routine bloods.
• Phone a haematologist or (ideally) the nearest haemophiliac service. Usually they will take blood for you (ask the haematologist where the nearest service is).
• Use paediatric bottles from the paediatrics ward to minimize the amount of blood needed.
• Never use a vacutainer; its 18 gauge needle is too big. Use the smallest possible needle or blue butterfly on small veins. Knuckle veins can be useful.
• Never use a tourniquet. It causes excessive bruising and occasionally major bleeds from pressure trauma to blood vessels. If you need pressure to find a vein, very gently inflate a blood pressure cuff, but release the pressure as soon as you are in the vein, or you will cause major bruising.
• Never give or prescribe drugs IM.
• Always use standard precautions for taking blood samples. Nearly all UK haemophiliac adults have Hep C, and about two-thirds have HIV.
• Always alert the lab to the haemophiliac status of patient and their hepatitis/HIV status.
• Tell patients why you are taking blood and that you are taking care to avoid any unnecessary tests. These patients are often loathe to have more blood taken.

For theatre

• Do a full clotting screen (INR, bleeding time, APTT, fibrinogen) pre-operatively and a screen for antibodies. Liaise with the haematologist. Any deficiency of factors VIII or IX must be corrected before theatre. If the deficiency is corrected, the patient can be treated like other patients post-operatively, except:
  • Factor VIII levels should be tested post-operatively twice per day (factor IX levels once per day). Make sure the first level is taken *before* the patient is bathed and the wound dressed.
  • Delay suture removal beyond the usual 10 days, as haemophiliacs are prone to bleeding about this time. Get senior advice.

HIV/AIDS

It goes without saying that these patients need special care. They face both death and stigma. You face potentially dangerous needlestick injuries. Time, care and an honest, open approach are essential.

Taking blood

• It is completely fine to touch HIV/AIDS patients without gloves just about anywhere – just not in a major artery! It is really awful for such patients if health professionals are scared to treat them normally.

• However, do always wear gloves when taking blood. Always have plenty of space for your tray and sharps. Use a nursing trolley if possible and have separate cardboard trays for sharps.

• Don't do things in a hurry. Leave plenty of time for procedures and explanations.

• Label blood samples with high risk stickies (not in front of the patient). These are available from the labs if they are not already on your ward. It is your responsibility if a lab worker contracts HIV from an unlabelled sample.

• Use two specimen bags for high risk samples.

• Always warn theatre staff if a patient has HIV or AIDS.

• Treat oral *Candida* with nystatin lozenges (mild) or ketoconazole/miconazole (see the *BNF*).

• Be aware that HIV/AIDS patients may suffer from depression and may consider suicide. Consider referring to the psychiatrists or social workers. Discuss the patient with the nursing staff—and the patient, of course!

• AIDS patients may suffer from multiple serious medical problems which may require urgent or aggressive therapy. Common problems include: fever, atypical pneumonia, diarrhoea, skin sores, and drug reactions. For reasons that are as yet poorly understood, allergies are much more common in patients with AIDS. If you find yourself looking after an AIDS patient in a general ward, get expert advice from infectious disease staff.

• If necessary, reassure non-medical ward staff that they cannot catch HIV from an AIDS patient, so that they don't emit an aura of apprehension that the patient will quickly detect.

HIV testing

Patients need counselling and preparation for HIV tests. Discuss doing HIV tests with seniors; they can advise you on hospital policy. The ward's social worker may be able to help you with this.

• Explain HIV/AIDS. Being HIV-positive is not the same thing as having AIDS. At present 50% of asymptomatic HIV-positive patients get AIDS after 10 years.

• Explain the benefits of the test. If the patient is HIV-positive, you can monitor T cell function, treat infection better, and he or she can practise safe sex and protect their partner. 24-hour support is available for people with HIV.

• Explain the problems of the test. Some life insurance companies may discriminate against you (this is being phased out). A way around this is to get tested anonymously at an STD clinic.

• Arrange with a virologist to have the blood tested as soon as possible (so the patient is not stewing for days).

• Label the sample carefully and take all precautions when taking it.

• Tell the patient at what time the result will be back. If there is any delay, let the patient know and reassure them that it is not due to their sample being infected.

Jehovah's Witnesses/ Christian Scientists

• As with any person, you cannot force a Jehovah's Witness or Christian Scientist to accept treatment (e.g. a blood transfusion). Make sure they sign a statement acknowledging refusal of treatment. Most hospitals have policy documents and suitable consent or exemption forms. Discuss the case with your seniors.

• In an emergency, you can legally instigate treatment to save someone's life unless it is clear that the patient has given an informed refusal of that treatment which remains in force. Again, get nursing and senior advice and, if necessary, advice from your defence organization.

Pregnant women

• Get senior advice about X-rays in pregancy (see p. 173). Make sure you notify the radiologist that the patient is pregnant – write it clearly on the form and preferably speak to the radiologist yourself.

• Always ask women of child-bearing age the date of their LMP and whether or not they are likely to be pregnant.

• Pregnant women have hyperdynamic, volume-expanded circulations. Their JVPs are usually slightly raised. This is OK, but it also means that they can lose a lot of blood before they exhibit signs of hypovolaemia.

• Most drugs are potentially toxic. Make sure you know the trimester and always get senior or pharmacist advice before prescribing.

• Fetuses are like enormous tumours. They consume folate, iron, Ca and other vitamins that would normally go to the mother. Ensure that pregnant women have adequate nutrition and supplement if necessary.

• Be wary of pregnant women with abdominal pain. Organs such as the appendix get displaced, and inflammation can present in bizarre ways. For example, appendicitis may present as chest pain if it irritates the diaphragm. Always seek senior advice. Consider notifying an obstetrician.

Sickle cell anaemia

Be alert to sickle cell anaemia in any black, Arabic, Indian or Mediterranean patient within the UK with acute pain in the spine, joints, chest or abdomen. Within the UK, all patients of African descent need a sickling test before surgery. Heterozygous patients are only likely to suffer severe symptoms when hypoxic, as may occur during anaesthesia or at high altitudes. However, in homozygous patients, sickling crises are precipitated by hypoxia, infection, cold and other common stressors. Sickling crises can develop with alarming rapidity and can be fatal without prompt treatment. The patient will often know when they are going into crisis.

1 Symptoms of a sickle crisis include severe bone pain, acute abdominal pain, SOB and neurological symptoms such as fits and cranial nerve palsies.

2 Basic management includes prompt **analgesia** (pethidine 100–200 mg IM 2 hourly as required), O_2 therapy, **rehydration** (ensure fluid intake of at least 3 l/day) and **antibiotics** if

Table 10.2 Anti-inflammatory steroid equivalent doses.

Steroid	Dose
Dexamethasone and betamethasone	0.75 mg
Methylprednisolone and triamcinolone	4 mg
Prednisolone	5 mg
Hydrocortisone	20 mg

pyrexial or evidence of infection. Make sure the patient is warm. Seek urgent, expert help especially if they do not improve quickly—these patients can deteriorate within hours!. Lung involvement is particularly worrying.

3 Investigations: the patient will need urgent IV access and baseline bloods, cross-match, FBC, reticulocyte count and film, blood cultures, MSU and chest X-ray. Include ABGs if there is any CXR-shadowing, respiratory symptoms or infection). Measure Hb daily.

4 If the patient needs surgery, seek specialist anaesthetic advice.

The steroid patient

Patients on steroids are vulnerable to infection and other side effects, and may require additional steroid cover while ill. Steroids affect the immune system, fluid balance, carbohydrate, lipid and protein metabolism. Anti-inflammatory steroid equivalent doses are shown in Table 10.2.

Side effects of steroids

Mineralocorticoid
Na and water retention, hypertension
Hypokalaemia

Glucocorticoid
Diabetes
Changes in fat distribution
Changes in protein mobilization: osteoporosis, skin atrophy, striae, muscle wasting, delayed wound healing

Mental changes
These occur in most patients. They vary from subtle changes to frank paranoid psychosis. Warn the patient (and relatives and friends!) that they may become easily irritable or 'difficult' and that they should inform the doctor if this causes problems. Initial euphoria and increased appetite are common

Infection
Candida infection: oesophageal (dysphagia) or vaginal (itching)

continued

Disseminated viral infection: measles, varicella zoster and herpes zoster
Bacterial infection. The inflammatory response is suppressed hence late presentation and rapid systemic spread of infection. Be alert to the 'silent' abdomen, septicaemia and TB

Others
Peptic ulceration: severe dyspepsia is common although the link to ulceration is less well understood
Acne is common
Withdrawal reactions (see below)

Management of the ill patient on steroids

Illness (acute stress, especially surgery or infection) increases steroid requirements. Decide if your patient needs additional steroids or not. Prescribe hydrocortisone 25–100 mg tds (or equivalent) in addition to existing steroid dose if required. See p. 187 for surgical steroid cover. Always be aware of 'silent' infections in a patient on high dose steroids (see side effects).

Treating common side effects

1 *Candida* infection. Prescribe nystatin lozenges or miconazole oral gel for oral/oesophageal infection, and clotrimazole (Canesten) cream/vaginal pessaries for vaginal infection. Fluconazole 50 mg PO daily is useful as prophylaxis for high dose steroids.
2 If the patient is known to suffer from cold sores or shingles, tell the patient to start high dose acyclovir at the earliest sign of recurrence.
3 Heartburn. Prescribe ranitidine 150 mg nocte or equivalent.

Withdrawal of steroid therapy

The longer the patient has been on steroids, the more gradual the reduction of steroids needs to be. Abrupt withdrawal may cause acute adrenal insufficiency or Addisonian crisis. Therapy for longer than 2 weeks can lead to adrenal suppression.

You can reduce steroids from high doses by 5–10 mg of prednisolone (or equivalent)/week until you reach the equivalent of 10 mg prednisolone/day. Thereafter, reduce by 2.5 mg/week until you reach 5 mg/day. After this, the rate of reduction depends on the preceding length of therapy. If this was greater than 3 months, reduce slowly, e.g. by 1–2 mg/week.

Withdrawal reactions

Addisonian crisis (hypotension, dehydration, hyperkalaemia, hyponatraemia), arthralgia, conjunctivitis, mood change, rhinitis, skin rashes – itchy nodules or acne, weight loss. Morning irritability can be prevented by taking the daily dose bd.

Chapter 11: Approach to the medical patient

A major task during medical house jobs is clerking patients. This section provides an approach to history and examination of the medical patient, and how to optimize your time in getting to know the patient and in getting a feel for their problems.

In general, with the introduction of shift work, you may find yourself looking after a patient you did not admit and do not know. It is well worth the effort to re-clerk these patients as soon as possible. It takes much less time than you think and will allow you to develop a better relationship with the patient. While your night-shift colleagues are unlikely to miss an obvious sign, it is remarkable how much more information is yielded by a history taken in the light of day.

An approach to history taking comprises two essential parts, which enable management to be tailored to the individual patient and his or her disease:

1 Getting to know the patient (the person and their medical background).
2 Getting to know the disease (the presenting problem).

Getting to know the patient as a person

Patient ID — age, sex, etc.
Work.
Lives with.
Social support — family, friends, finances.

Mobility.
Home help.
Problems as perceived by the patient: worries, fears.

The medical background

Past medical history.
Past surgical history.
What operations and any anaesthetic complications?
Allergies, drug history.
Family history.

Getting to know the disease

Presenting complaints. Identify as clearly as possible the reason for the patient presenting now and think of the possible causes for the symptoms so that you establish an early ranked differential diagnosis. Never take a history blindly. Always be aware of the diagnostic possibilities based on the background and the presenting complaint so that you ask questions that strengthen or refute a specific possibility. At this stage it is useful to stop, think and construct a ranked differential diagnosis before the next phase of the history taking.

The present history. This is what the patient tells you about their present illness. Listen carefully and ask clarifying questions. Attempt to live the patient's life from the onset of the symptoms so that you become aware of important details that will refine your differential diagnosis. At the end of this, try to refine your differential diagnosis and identify those features of the most likely diseases that have emerged thus far. Ask about these features now – *the specific directed enquiry*, and write down your differential diagnosis and problem list before the examination.

The systematic (or functional) enquiry. This is the least useful part of the history. While it provides a convenient list of symptoms, it encourages thoughtless history taking that overworked junior doctors don't need! It should therefore be left until last but not omitted. For the detailed list of symptoms see the outline below.

The examination

The same general examination for all patients should be followed by a directed systemic examination, based on the diagnostic possibilities elicited in your history. For example, you would make a careful check for signs of SBE in a patient with a history of valvular heart disease and recent decrease in exercise tolerance. Note the important negative findings, e.g. no splinter haemorrhages, no vasculitic skin lesions, no splenomegaly. Fully document your findings.

We provide an outline of the general and systematic examination of the medical patient on p. 115. While it is structured in the order for 'routine' examination, few patients are 'routine', and you should examine some systems in more detail according to your differential diagnosis.

Summing up

At the end of your history and examination, it is a good idea to sum-up for presenting on ward rounds.
1 Patient ID and salient medical background. (Mention only that which is pertinent to the present problem.)
2 Presenting complaint.
3 Current problems – medical, pharmacological, social.
4 Investigations.
5 Plan for discharge – how the team is going about solving the patient's problems and the likely time of discharge from hospital.

History and examination

Figures 11.1 & 11.2 provide an outline of the above approach to history and examination. Re-type and photocopy if you want.

Clinical stalemate

Your patient sits in bed day after day, and no progress is made. What do you do?
1 Decide if the patient is sick or not, and getting better or getting sicker day by day. Sometimes you should let well alone.
2 If the patient is ill or getting worse, then rapidly identify the main problems and make a management plan, e.g. is the renal function, mental state or pulmonary function deteriorating?
3 Having addressed obvious problems, review the case. It can be helpful to 're-clerk' the patient, especially as this clerking will have the benefit of hind-

Getting to know the patient as a person

Patient ID—age, sex, etc.

Work .... Mobility ....

Lives with .... Home help ....

Social support— Problems as perceived by the patient,

family, friends .... worries, fears ....

Finances ....

The medical background

Past medical history

1 CVS—IHD, rheumatic fever, hypertension, other ....

2 RS—asthma, smoker, TB, exposure to irritants ....

3 Diabetes, thyroid disease, other medical illnesses ....

Past surgical history

What operations ....

Any anaesthetic complications ....

Drug history and allergies

Current medication ....

Relevant past medication ....

Allergies ....

Family history ....

Hobbies and pets ....

Getting to know the disease

Presenting complaint/s ....

....

(STOP—THINK—CONSTRUCT A RANKED DIFFERENTIAL DIAGNOSIS)

The present history and the specific directed enquiry

(What the patient tells you about their illness and directed questions to define the differential.)

Systematic (or functional) enquiry

1 General—loss of appetite, loss of weight, fever, night sweats, any lumps, itch and rashes.

2 CVS/RS—chest pain, dyspnoea, orthopnoea, PND, cough, haemoptysis, sputum, ankle oedema, intermittent claudication

3 GIT—dyspepsia, nausea, vomiting, diarrhoea, change in bowel habit, blood or mucus PR.

4 GU—dysuria, frequency, urgency, nocturia, haematuria, polyuria, incontinence.

5 Gynaecology—vaginal discharge, menses, first day of last period (LMP), menarche, menopause, pregnancy.

6 CNS—fits, blackouts, headaches, visual disturbances, sensory disturbances, weakness/paralysis, falls, loss of hearing. Higher mental function.

7 MSK/skin—joint pain/swelling, stiffness.

Refined differential diagnosis

....

....

Fig. 11.1 Approach to history taking.

Examination

In order of examination

1 Appearance. Does the patient look ill? General nutrition
2 Temperature

Working up the arm:

3 Hands, nails
4 Pulse
5 Respiratory rate
6 While doing the above, consider evidence of endocrine disease (pituitary, thyroid, Addisons), or Paget's: body hair, skin pigmentation, skin lesions
7 BP
8 Eyes–pallor, jaundice
9 Mouth and tongue–cyanosis, smooth or furred tongue, any lesions?
10 Examine the neck–nodes, goitre

CVS examination with patient at 45°:

11 JVP and cartoid pulses
12 Praecordium–inspect, palpate, auscultate
13 Sacral oedema? Ankle oedema?

RS examination with patient at 90°:

14 Chest–inspect, palpate (trachea, expansion), auscultate
15 Breasts and axillary nodes

GIT examination with patient lying flat:

16 Abdomen–inspect, palpate (tenderness, visceromegaly), auscultate (bowel sounds)

Legs:

17 Swelling, pulses

CNS examination:

The detail of this examination will depend on the differential diagnosis. The essentials include:

18 Cranial nerves–pupil responses; fundi; corneal reflexes; 'Open your mouth; stick out your tongue; show me your teeth; shut your eyes tightly; raise your eyebrows; shrug your shoulders'
19 Peripheral nerves and motor function–wasting; sensation (vibration, light touch); tone; power; gait
20 Speech and higher mental functions
21 Do PR and FOB test. Consider PV
22 Dipstick urine and consider microscopy
23 Summarize findings and list your plan for solving the patient's problems:
   • Patient ID and salient medical background
   • Presenting complaint/s ....

   • Current problem/s ....

   • Investigations ....

   • Plan for discharge ....

Fig. 11.2 Approach to examination.

sight, and the use of previous notes, the patient's drug chart, etc.

Main complaint
History of main complaint
PMH
Drugs, allergies, habits, travel, etc.

4 Repeat a complete examination. Like the history, the examination will benefit from hindsight and recent investigation results. Examine test results critically – are they reliable or spurious? Are they up to date?

5 Formulate now a list of problems, differential diagnoses, and investigations to be requested. You may not come up with blinding new answers immediately, but you will know the case a lot better, and you will avoid the embarrassment of having overlooked key pieces of information in the history, examination and investigations.

6 Now write a summary in the notes of your findings at this stage. If appropriate, use tables for important serial data.

Preparing patients for medical procedures

During your house job you will prepare patients for many different procedures. This section explains what needs to be done and what complications to expect. It is important to realize that while most procedures are routine for you, they are usually frightening for patients. Probably the scariest thing is not knowing what will happen next, so lots of information can make a big difference. A list of patients' common concerns about procedures includes:

1 What does the procedure entail?
2 Why are they having this done?
3 How long will the procedure take?

4 Do they need a general anaesthetic?
5 Will the procedure be painful?
6 What should they do if they have pain or other symptoms after the procedure?
7 When can they eat/drink/drive/talk/have sex?
8 Will they have any scars/permanent after-effects?
9 Who is doing the procedure?

Upper gastrointestinal endoscopy

Preparation

1 Consent.
2 NBM for 4 hours. If you suspect gastric outlet obstruction, allow only water for 8 hours and NBM for 4 hours.
3 FBC and INR (in case of biopsy).
4 Insert cannula (usually 23 G, although 21 G sometimes suffices) in the arm that will make endoscopic manoeuvring easiest (usually the right arm).
5 Barium can block the suction channel of the endoscope, so delay for 24 hours following upper GI barium studies.

Consider telling the patient

1 What endoscopy is and why they are having it.
2 That the procedure takes about 5–10 minutes, although it may seem longer.
3 During the procedure, they will be given IV sedation, but not a general anaesthetic, to make them drowsy. They shouldn't drive until the following day. Also, their throat will be sprayed with local anaesthetic so that they won't feel the endoscope too much.
4 An endoscope (tube) the thickness of a little finger is passed into the food pipe

and into the stomach. It is uncomfortable but not painful.

5 The doctor might take a tiny sample of the inside of the gullet or stomach to examine under a microscope. This is painless.

6 The patient can eat and drink after the local anaesthetic has worn off, which should take about half an hour. They might have a sore throat which should get better within 1–2 days.

Complications

1 Transient sore throat and possible numbness.

2 Rarely oesophageal perforation (<1 in 1000).

3 Mild bleeding (and rarely haemorrhage) following a biopsy.

Colonoscopy

Preparation

1 Consent.

2 Low residue diet for 36 hours and fluids only for 12 hours before the procedure.

3 Two Picolax sachets (sodium picosulphate and magnesium citrate) or equivalent 24 hours before the procedure. Use one sachet for frail, elderly patients. Do not give to patients with inflamed colonic mucosa (UC, Crohn's, etc.).

Consider telling the patient

1 What colonoscopy is (a way of looking directly at the bowel) and why they are having it.

2 Warn that Picolax causes explosive diarrhoea. They need to drink plenty of clear fluids to maintain hydration (2–3 litres/day: three to four jugs of squash).

3 IV sedation is given that will make them drowsy, but it is not a general anaesthetic (usually).

4 A flexible tube is passed into their back passage.

5 The whole thing takes about 20–30 minutes, and the patient can go home accompanied as soon as the sedation has worn off – usually in about 2 hours. They shouldn't drive until the following day.

Complications

1 Mild abdominal discomfort during and after the procedure is common due to a small amount of gas that is pumped in to aid vision through the colonoscope during the procedure.

2 Incomplete examination, requiring a second examination or barium enema, occurs in about 10% of cases.

3 Perforation occurs about 1 in 500, more commonly in acute colitis or extensive diverticulosis. If this unlikely event happens, the person usually will need to have their bowel repaired under a general anaesthetic.

4 Serious haemorrhage post-biopsy or polypectomy is rare.

Flexible sigmoidoscopy

Preparation

Two phosphate enemas.

Explanation as for colonoscopy except sedation is not usually required.

Liver biopsy

Preparation

1 Consent.
2 Bloods: FBC−Hb and platelets, INR and APTT, liver biochemistry and G&S.
3 Abdominal US advisable to check anatomy (ask the person performing the procedure).
4 Mild pre-med, such as pethidine (50 mg) and prochlorperazine (12.5 mg). Temazepam (10 mg) can also be given if the patient is not at risk of hepatic failure or jaundiced.
5 IV access with at least a green cannula.

Consider telling the patient

1 What a liver biopsy is and why they need one.
2 The procedure is performed on the ward or in an operating theatre. The biopsy itself is very quick (a few seconds) but the whole procedure might take up to 30 minutes−and may seem longer than this. They will have to stay in hospital overnight.
3 The procedure does not usually involve heavy sedation or a general anaesthetic.
4 The site of the biopsy is on the patient's right side, between the 8th and 10th ribs. The patient will need to help by holding their breath during the biopsy.

Complications

1 Shoulder tip or local abdominal pain for a few hours (up to 2 days) is common but relieved by paracetamol 1 g 4–6-hourly.
2 Bleeding possibly requiring transfusion (about 1 in 50).
3 Infection, abscess, pneumothorax (rarely requiring drainage) and biliary peritonitis are uncommon (<1 : 100).

Following the procedure

1 The patient should lie on their right side for at least 2 hours and remain in bed (absolute bedrest) overnight.
2 Observations: BP and pulse every 15 minutes for 1 hour, then every 30 minutes for 2 hours, then hourly for 6 hours. Ask to be informed if the BP falls (>15 mmHg) or if the pulse starts rising (>15 bpm).
3 Ensure that an IV line is secure and that analgesia is written up (ask the operator which they prefer).
4 Check the patient 4 and 8 hours following the biopsy for pain and vital signs.

Pacemaker insertion

Preparation

1 Informed consent
2 FBC and INR.

Consider telling the patient

1 What a pacemaker is and why they need one.
2 A very small wire is threaded via a large vein (the subclavian) into one of the chambers of the heart under X-ray screening. The wire is gently inserted into the wall of the heart. The other end of the wire is connected to a machine called a pacemaker that generates heart beats, which is placed into a small pocket fashioned in the fatty tissues of

the chest. Its battery will not run out! The pacemaker causes a small lump under the skin on the upper thorax, but nowadays the generators are so small these are hardly noticeable.

3 The procedure is performed under local anaesthetic, sometimes with mild sedation.

4 The procedure is mostly painless. It takes 30–60 minutes.

5 In future, the patient will need to carry a card that says they are fitted with a permanent pacemaker, in case they ever need emergency treatment. A Medicalert bracelet is recommended.

6 Caution in pregnancy, as X-ray screening is used during the procedure.

Complications

1 As for central line placement – pneumothorax, bleeding.

2 Dislodgement of the wire leading to pacing failure. Electrical faults are uncommon.

Renal biopsy

Preparation

1 Consent.

2 Bloods: FBC–Hb and platelets, INR, G&S.

3 Abdominal US is essential to check that two kidneys are present.

4 Mild pre-med, such as pethidine (50 mg IM) and prochlorperazine (12.5 mg IM).

5 IV access with at least a green cannula.

Consider telling the patient

1 What a renal biopsy is and why they need one.

2 The procedure is usually done in theatre and takes a few minutes. Sedation is usually required (but not a general anaesthetic).

3 The biopsy is taken through the left or right flank. The patient will need to hold their breath briefly during the biopsy.

4 The patient should drink a lot of fluids after the biopsy, to flush the kidneys and avoid renal colic.

Complications

1 Local pain (prescribe analgesia) and mild haematuria are common.

2 Haemorrhage requiring transfusion is less common (about 1 in 30–60). Surgical intervention for massive haemorrhage is rare.

3 Renal colic from clots may occur.

Following the procedure

1 Patient should lie on the side of the biopsy for at least 2 hours and remain in bed (absolute bedrest) overnight.

2 Observation: BP and pulse every 15 minutes for 1 hour, then every 30 minutes for 2 hours, then hourly for 6 hours. Ask to be informed if the BP falls (>15 mmHg) or if the pulse starts rising (>15 bpm).

3 Check for gross haematuria.

4 Ensure IV access is OK and that good analgesia is written up.

5 Check on the patient 4 and 8 hours following the biopsy for pain, unstable vital signs and gross haematuria or bleeding.

Specialist referrals and investigating the medical case

Most consultants have their own pet investigations. Be guided by ward protocols, but ask someone if you do not understand the rationale for a particular investigation. Protocols often become outdated and nobody takes the time to inform the House Officer.

If a patient is unwell enough to be admitted, you should have the following results to hand:
1 Weight.
2 T.
3 BP.
4 Urine dipstick.
5 FBC and ESR.
6 Biochemistry – at least U&E.
When indicated:
7 CXR.
8 ECG.

Below, we provide a list of further investigations to anticipate, listed under system headings for commonly encountered pathologies. In addition, these are a useful checklist when making specialist referrals. You will greatly impress the visiting consultant if you have useful results to hand. If in doubt, bleep their House Officer to discover which investigations are the flavour of the month!

Cardiology

Essential investigations before referral to a cardiologist include ECG and rhythm strip and CXR. In specific situations, see below.

Suspected acute MI

1 Serial ECGs (three consecutive days).
2 Serial serum cardiac enzymes (some hospitals now offer CK-MB assay which, when taken about 12 hours after the onset of pain, offers a more specific and sensitive marker of MI).

IHD

1 Serum cholesterol and triglycerides.
2 Formal blood sugar (ward test is not good enough).

Heart failure (recent onset)

1 ECHO: urgent if there are murmurs of aortic valve disease or you suspect SBE (consider transoesophageal ECHO if local expertise available) or pericardial disease.

Hypertension

1 Cholesterol and triglycerides.
2 MSU for MC&S if blood or protein on urinary dipstick.
3 Ensure there is a recent record of an ECG, CXR and serum biochemistry.
4 US of the kidneys if symptoms are suggestive of clinical renal disease (history of nephritis, renal problems in childhood, family history of renal disease) or sudden onset or poorly controlled BP.

SBE

1 Blood cultures; at least three sets.
2 Rh factor.
3 Urine dipstick and microscopy.
4 Blood film, serum haptoglobins and urinary haemosiderin.

5 Consider transoesophageal ECHO.

Endocrinology

Except for DM, endocrine disorders are rare. Special tests are required according to the differential diagnosis before referral.

Diabetes mellitus

1 Flow chart the patients blood glucose readings and acetylated Hb (Hb-1Ac) if available
2 Renal function
  • Flow chart of creatinine levels.
  • 24 hour urine collection for creatinine clearance and protein.
3 Careful fundoscopy and ophthalmology referral.
4 Peripheral nerve examination.
5 Cholesterol and triglycerides.
6 ECG – have old ECGs to compare.
7 Arrange follow-up in diabetic clinic, arrange diabetic dietary advice by dietician, and involve the diabetic specialist nurse if available.

Investigation of Cushings

Consult a specialized lab for advice. Different labs prefer different tests.

Standard tests done in most labs include those listed below.
1 10 pm (not necessary to do it at midnight) and 9 am cortisol levels. The night level is usually lower than the morning level, but this diurnal cycle is lost in Cushings.
2 Shortened low-dose dexamethasone suppression test: 1 mg dexamethasone PO at 11 pm and measure the cortisol level in the morning around 9 am. In Cushings, the cortisol levels are not suppressed, whereas in pseudo-Cushings (e.g. depression, severe obesity and alcoholism), the cortisol level is suppressed.
3 High-dose dexamethasone suppression test: 0.5 mg dexamethasone 6-hourly for 48 hours. Next, measure the morning cortisol level at 24 and 48 hours. This suppresses cortisol levels in pituitary-dependent Cushing's disease, while it does not suppress cortisol levels in adrenal adenomas and ectopic ACTH.
4 Measure urinary-free cortisols (24 hour urine collections).
Note: the best evidence of Cushing's syndrome is the demonstration of loss of diurnal rhythm of cortisol secretion.

Investigations for phaeochromocytoma

Consult a specialized lab for advice. Different labs prefer different tests.

Standard tests done in most labs include those listed below.
1 Three 24 hour urine collections for catecholamines (adrenaline, noradrenaline metabolites (HMMA/VMA) or total metadrenalines). Requires a special urine bottle. Tell the patient to avoid vanilla, bananas and aspirin.
2 Consider CT or MRI scan of chest and abdomen (phaeo's can arise anywhere along the sympathetic chain), and/or special isotope (MIBG) scan, if the urine test is positive.

Thyroid disease

1 Hypothyroidism: raised TSH, low T_4.
2 Secondary hypothyroidism (rare): low T_4 and T_3 but TSH is not raised; look for pituitary failure.

3 Hyperthyroidism: suppressed TSH and raised T_4 or T_3. In 10% of patients with hyperthyroidism, only the T_3 is raised.

Gastroenterology

Always do a PR before referring to a gastroenterologist.

Gastroenterologists often request some unusual tests. Investigate according to the differential diagnosis.

Upper GI symptoms

1 Faecal occult bloods (×3).
2 Barium meal or gastroscopy.

GI bleeds (see pp. 59–61)

1 Cross-match.
2 Hb, platelets and INR.
3 Check LFTs, U&E.
4 Endoscopy.
5 Consider surgical consultation.

Chronic diarrhoea

1 Warm stool for MC&S including ova, cysts and parasites (×3), *Clostridium difficile* toxin and culture.
2 FBC (MCV).
3 LFTs (albumin).
4 Ca and phosphate.

Chronic lower GIT symptoms

1 Faecal occult bloods (×3).
2 Flexible sigmoidoscopy.
3 Consider barium enema or colonoscopy, depending on local expertise.
4 Consider a small bowel meal.
5 Consider other sources (e.g. GU tract) for symptoms.

Ascites of unknown origin

1 History of alcohol consumption.
2 Bloods for LFTs, hepatitis serology. Consider checking antimitochondrial antibodies (for primary biliary cirrhosis) and antismooth muscle cell antibodies (for chronic active hepatitis).
3 Aspirate the ascites (see p. 162). Reexamine following aspiration, especially the female pelvic organs. A PV is essential if the cause of ascites is unclear.
4 US the abdomen and pelvis (consider aspiration under US guidance if there is a small or loculated collection). US is most useful after aspiration. Specific points on US: Is the portal vein patent? Size and texture of liver and spleen? Porta hepatis nodes?
5 Consider a CT scan.
6 Consider a barium swallow or endoscopy for varices.
7 Consider peritoneoscopy—may be dependent on local expertise.
8 Consider a laparotomy.

Liver disease

1 INR, platelets, bleeding time.
2 Liver biochemistry.
3 Urine for bilirubin and urobilinogen.
4 Hepatitis screen—B and C (A if acute).
5 Iron/TIBC, caeruloplasmin, alpha-fetoprotein.
6 US abdomen.
7 Stool chart.
8 Consider liver biopsy.
9 Consider random alcohol level on this or next admission. MCV and GGT.

Haematology

Essential investigations before referral

include FBC, differential, film and ESR.

Suspected DIC

1 FDPs.
2 INR and APTT.
3 LFTs.
4 Urine dipstick and microscopy.
5 Blood cultures.
(DIC is not an end diagnosis – you must find the cause).

Anaemia (see p. 37)

1 Reticulocyte count +/− sickle cell status.
2 Serum bilirubin, LDH (a marker of haemolysis).
3 Iron studies, vitamin B_{12}, serum and red cell folate.
4 CRP, ESR.
5 Consider bone marrow biopsy.

Suspected paraprotein/myeloma

1 ESR and viscosity.
2 Serum and urine electrophoresis, urine collection for light chains (15% of patients have urinary light chains only).
3 Skeletal survey.
4 Bone marrow biopsy.

Neurology

A thorough history and examination are by far the most important things to do before referral.

Meningism

1 Do LP (see p. 158) if there are no signs of raised ICP (rising BP, papilloedema, depressed LOC).

- LP pressure.
- MC&S, cell count, xanthochromia.
- Consider Indian ink stains for *Cryptococcus*, ZN for AFBs, viral PCR.
- Glucose.
- Protein.

2 Consider serology for *Cryptococcus*, syphilis and viral causes of meningitis.
3 Consider CT scan head. If suspicious of raised ICP, do CT scan first.

Unexplained coma

Before referral you should:
1 Ensure that the patient's ABC are adequate.
2 Obtain a history from relatives, friends and GP, especially regarding possible drug overdose or recent travel abroad.
3 Do a secondary neurological examination for clues. The neurological exam would initially have been restricted to the Glasgow Coma Scale and hard localizing signs.
4 Have the following results clearly documented (if available):
- Blood glucose stick that was done immediately on admission.
- FBC, U&E, Ca, phosphate, blood glucose.
- Liver biochemistry.
- Urine dipstick and MC&S.
- ABGs and toxicology screen.

5 Arrange an urgent CT scan head +/− LP.
6 Send a serum sample for storage (serology).
Note: MRI scans are becoming a common investigation for neurology patients.

Renal medicine

Renal physicians rely heavily on bio-chemistry to manage their patients, so have a flow chart of the patient's U&E and creatinine results. Get their help *early* if a patient's renal function is deteriorating.

Renal failure/nephrotics/nephritics

1 BP.
2 Fresh urine for microscopy (do on ward) and send sample for MC&S.
3 Daily weights.
4 Fluid intake/output chart.
5 Serology.
- Virology: CMV, Hep B and C and HIV if candidate for haemodialysis/transplant (remember to counsel the patient).
- Bacteriology: VDRL and atypical serology.
- Immunology: CRP, Igs and serum electrophoresis, complement and autoantibodies; ANA intially, but also consider ANCA, anti-GBM and cryoglobulins.
6 Biochemistry: in addition to renal and hepatic indices request: Ca, total pro-tein, albumin, phosphate.
7 24-hour urine collection – protein and creatinine clearance.
8 Renal US – do early to exclude ob-struction, especially if the renal function is deteriorating.
9 Consider renal biopsy.

Renal biopsy (see p. 119)

Recurrent UTIs

1 BP, MSU.
2 Creatinine clearance.

3 Abdominal X-ray to look for calculi. Consider an IVU (looking for structural anomalies).
4 US kidneys (document the size).
5 Consider a micturating cystogram (reflux).
6 PR and proctoscopy.
7 PV and speculum.
8 Consider a urology referral.

Respiratory medicine

Essential investigations before referral to a respiratory physician are CXRs, ECGs and results of lung function tests and ABGs.

Pneumonia

1 CXR.
2 Sputum for MC&S, cytology and AFB.
3 Physiotherapy if bronchopneumonia or exacerbation of COAD – arrange ASAP. Physiotherapy is not indicated for lobar pneumonia.
4 ABGs are mandatory for any severe respiratory illness.
5 Send a serum sample for storage if you suspect an atypical pneumonia (*Legionella, Mycoplasma* etc).

If you suspect TB

1 Sputum for AFB. (A 5% saline nebu-lizer will encourage productive cough-ing if sputum is difficult to obtain.)
2 3× early morning specimens of urine for AFB.
3 Mantoux test (see p. 161).

Obstructive lung disease

1 Lung function tests pre- and post-bronchodilators.

Respiratory failure

1 ABGs and acid–base. (Bicarbonate is a useful indicator of chronic CO_2 retention.)

Pleural effusion

1 Send aspirate for:
   • Protein, LDH.
   • MC&S, AFBs and TB culture.
   • Cytology.
   • Glucose.
2 Consider pleural biopsy.
3 Consider tuberculin skin test.

Rheumatology

'Look, feel and move' all salient joints. FBC, ESR and CRP. X-rays of relevant joints.

Polyarthritis

1 Urate.
2 Fresh urine for microscopy.
3 X-ray affected joints.
4 CRP.
5 ASOT, serum sample for storage.
6 Latex fixation for Rheumatoid factor.
7 Auto-antibodies screen – ANAs.
8 Consider joint aspiration +/− synovial biopsy.

Chapter 12: Pain

This section is designed to help you deal with pain control on the general wards. The first section provides a general approach to pain control and summarizes commonly used analgesics, categorized by method of administration (inhalational, oral, IM/IV, etc). The boxed section is written by a pain relief specialist, giving an overview of the crucial and often overlooked aspects of pain control. Finally we provide tables for managing pain according to its severity and underlying clinical conditions.

Pain control

Pain control is critical to good clinical practice, yet it is often poorly managed and poorly understood. This section gives suggestions for dealing with acute pain that you are most likely to encounter on the wards. It is important to realize that while many of these suggestions apply also to chronic pain, do not be afraid to seek senior or specialist advice.

General

• When you are first presented with a patient in acute pain, you need to decide whether it is safe to treat the pain symptomatically, or whether you should further investigate its cause before masking the symptoms. Don't just treat pain – where possible, find the underlying cause!

• Analgesics are much more effective when used prophylactically. Frequent, mild analgesia may control pain much better than one-off hits of stronger preparations.

• Anticipate common side effects of analgesics, listed in Tables 12.2–12.4. Also be alert to idiosyncratic drug reactions such as rashes and blood dyscrasias.

• You will greatly alleviate acute physical pain by addressing the patient's fear and anxiety. Reassure the patient that the pain can and will be lessened. Next, prescribe an appropriate analgesic (see Tables 12.5 and 12.6).

Specific analgesics

Inhaled drugs (see Table 12.1)

Entonox (50% nitrous oxide, 50% oxygen).

Oral drugs

Paracetamol (see Table 12.2)

Non-steroidal anti-inflammatory drugs (see Table 12.3)

• Aspirin - use of eneteric-coated preparations reduces dyspepsia.
• Naproxen—low incidence of side effects, highly effective for inflammatory pain.

Crucial and often overlooked aspects of pain control

There are two types of pain: acute and chronic. Furthermore, each type of pain has two components: physical (sensory or 'stimulus-dependent') and emotional (Fig. 12.1). In addition, some pain cannot be reduced to physical or emotional components. This is known as 'stimulus-independent' pain. Finally, the relative importance of each component can change, so each patient's pain needs to be assessed daily. Bear in mind that the emotional component is often missed, but may be the most significant contributing factor.

Physical (stimulus-dependent) and stimulus-independent pain

In both acute and chronic pain, the stimulus and the response may not always be

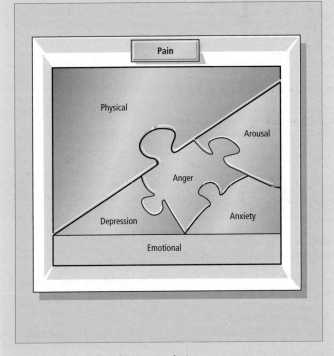

Fig. 12.1 Emotional and physical components of pain.

continued on p. 128

directly related. There is often background pain independent of the stimulus. Indeed, in chronic pain there may be no relationship between the stimulus and the pain perceived. This 'stimulus-independent' pain is often referred to as neuropathic pain, may be strongly affected by emotion (but not necessarily) and can be extremely difficult to treat. Such pain requires a different approach than stimulus-dependent pain. An example of this is the pain of post-herpetic neuralgia. These patients have altered pain perception: they may be numb to a pinprick but find light touch extremely painful. The most successful treatment for this pain is antidepressants, typifying the enigma of the neuropathic component of pain.

Emotional component of pain

There are four basic mood factors: arousal or awareness, anxiety, unhappiness or depression and anger (Fig. 12.1). The experience of pain is affected – and often heightened – by these different factors.

In *acute pain*, fear and anxiety heightens pain perception. These are usually reduced by treatment with regular pain-killers together with reassurance that pain is to be expected and can be controlled. Occasionally, the emotional response is so intense that it is necessary to use a sedative such as midazolam. For example, arousal (awareness) during procedures is very unpleasant. In endoscopy, opiates are given in combination with sedatives (e.g. pethidine and midazolam) thus dealing with both the physical and emotional responses to the stimuli.

In *chronic pain*, the emotional response can include chronic anxiety, depression and anger or frustration, to varying degrees. The clinical significance of these responses needs to be identified and treated. Patients with chronic pain are often angry that the medical profession cannot cure them and may inadvertently vent their frustration on junior staff. Such patients are best referred for treatment at the local pain clinic. Chronic pain patients are professional patients and need professional help!

• Diclofenac - see naproxen.
• Diflusinal - see naproxen. Longer half life allows for twice daily doses.
• Ibuprofen - fewer side effects than other NSAIDs though less anti-inflammatory activity.
• Tenoxicam - similar to naproxen. Long half life allows once daily administration.

Opiates (oral)

For pros and cons, see Table 12.4 for IM/IV opiates.

• Codeine - mild to moderate analgesia. High incidence of constipation and drowsiness. N&V are unusual.
• Dihydrocodeine - similar to codeine.
• Morphine (oral) - usually prescribed as slow release preparation. Used for chronic pain in terminally ill patients. High doses are often required as tolerance (tachyphylaxis) develops quite rapidly.

Table 12.1 Entonox (50% nitrous oxide and 50% oxygen).

Pros	Cons
Excellent for one-off or routine painful procedures where the stimulus and response are predictable	Does not work in all patients
Simple, fast and relatively safe	It cannot be used continuously or excessively because it causes bone marrow depression in a dose-dependent manner

Note: Never strap the mask in place; you may suffocate the patient. The patient should hold the mask.

Table 12.2 Paracetamol.

Pros	Cons
Very few side effects Useful for mild pain	Hepatotoxic in overdose

Table 12.3 Non-steroidal anti-inflammatory drugs (NSAIDs).

Pros	Cons
Excellent for treating pain associated with inflammation	NSAIDs share many side effects, commonly dyspepsia and nausea
Antipyretic	Occasional GI bleeding/ulceration, diarrhoea
The use of ulcer prophylactic drugs (e.g. ranitidine) has made the use of NSAIDs safer	Rarely hypersensitivity reactions (angio-oedema, urticaria, bronchospasm); headache; dizziness; vertigo; tinnitus; renal failure
	Caution in the elderly or if volume depleted (low GFR)
	There is considerable variability in individual patient response to a particular drug

IM/IV opiates

Bolus injection

• This involves slow IV injection over 2–3 minutes.
• Morphine - most commonly used, standard opiate for bad pain (see Table 12.5).
• Pethidine – much weaker analgesic properties than morphine. Most often used as pain prophylaxis for procedures.
• Diamorphine – similar analgesic properties as morphine. 5 mg is equivalent to 10 mg of morphine. It is more soluble than morphine, so easier for SC infusions.
• Papaveretum – mixture of morphine, codeine and papaverine. Most com-

Table 12.4 IM/IV opiates.

Pros	Cons
Potent analgesics Excellent for pain relief in the terminally ill Side effects tend to be dose dependent though there is variability between individual patients Naloxone is a highly effective antidote for opiate overdose (hypotension, respiratory depression). Give in incremental doses of 100–200 µg IV every 2 minutes. Beware of overtreating and throwing the patient into severe pain.	Opiates share many side effects, commonly nausea, vomiting, constipation and drowsiness. Respiratory depression and hypotension at higher doses An anti-emetic is usually required Addictive

monly used by anaesthetists for peri-operative analgesia.

Infusions (SC and PCA)

Morphine and diamorphine are commonly given as continuous infusions, particularly post-op or in the terminally ill. They can be administered as SC, continuous infusions or can be PCA. Different hospitals use different pumps; ask nursing and medical colleagues how to set up opiate infusions for your patients. Also consult the *BNF* and see p. 96.

Opiate antidote

Naloxone is a highly effective antidote for opiate overdose (small pupils, hypotension, respiratory depression). Give in incremental doses of 100–200 µg IV every 2 minutes. Beware of overtreating; analgesia may be reversed.

Other

Nerve blockades are rarely given by junior House Officers. The technique for local blockade is described on p. 157. Epidural and spinal blockades are specialist procedures.

TENS (transcutaneous electrical nerve stimulation).

Acupuncture can be very effective for certain types of pain.

Pain control by severity and underlying condition

It is useful to categorize the patient's pain as mild, moderate or severe, and to become familiar with the use of two or three preparations in each category. Our favourite analgesics are listed in Tables 12.5 and 12.6.

Hints

• Many of the compound analgesics contain small doses of codeine or other opiate analgesics. The *BNF* reports that these doses are of little clinical benefit

Table 12.5 Recommended analgesics for different levels of pain.

Mild pain
1 Paracetamol 500–1000 mg 4–6-hourly. Max dose in 24 hours is 4 g
2 Aspirin 300–900 mg 4–6-hourly. Max dose in 24 hours is 4 g. Use of enteric coated tablets is recommended to reduce dyspepsia
3 Ibuprofen 400–600 mg 8-hourly. Max dose is 2.4 g daily

Moderate pain
1 Co-dydramol contains paracetamol (500 mg) and dihydrocodeine (10 mg) in each tablet Dose 1–2 tablets 4–6 hourly. Max 8 tablets daily. Remedeine contains paracetamol plus dihydrocodeine in 20 or 30 mg strengths
2 NSAIDs: Diclofenac 75–150 mg PO daily in 2 divided doses; should be taken with food. Dose by IM injection: 75 mg once daily for a max of 2 days. (Max dose 150 mg daily by any route)
3 Codeine 30–60 mg PO/IM 4-hourly. Max dose 240 mg daily. Constipation is common so prescribe a prophylactic laxative (see p. 46)

Severe pain
1 Morphine sulphate 10 mg IM 4-hourly or 2–5 mg IV 4-hourly. (Use 15 mg IM for heavier, well-muscled patients)
2 Diamorphine 5 mg SC/IM 4-hourly or 0.5–2.5 mg/hour IV/SC as an infusion. (Use up to 10 mg IM/SC for heavier, muscular patients)
3 Pethidine 25–100 mg IV/IM/SC repeated after 4 hours. Max dose in 24 hours is 400 mg. Opiates are usually administered with a prophylactic anti-emetic such as prochlorperazine (10 mg PO, 30 minutes before giving the opiate, or 12.5 mg IM)

Table 12.6 Clinical conditions and commonly used analgesics.

Simple headache	Paracetamol
Severe post-op pain	Morphine, pethidine or papaveretum (IM/PO)
Colicky abdominal pain	Hyoscine butylbromide (Buscopan; an antimuscarinic) (PO/IV/IM)
Renal colic	Diclofenac (PO/IM)
Acute MI	Morphine or diamorphine (slow IV injection)
Pleuritic pain	NSAID, e.g. naproxen or diclofenac
Bone pain from metastases	Slow release oral morphine plus NSAIDs
Sciatica	Co-dydramol (mild pain), diclofenac or naproxen (severe pain)
Phantom limb pain	Meprobamate or carbamazepine (consult pain relief clinic)
Diabetic neuropathy	Carbamazepine (consult pain relief clinic)

whilst having the potential side effects of opiates. However, some patients swear by them and will only be happy if these are prescribed for their ailment. Common examples are Co-proxamol (paracetamol 325 mg plus dextropropoxyphene 32.5 mg) and Co-codamol (paracetamol 500 mg and codeine phosphate 8 mg).

• Ward stocks of compound analgesics may be limited to one or two brands you are not familiar with. Nursing staff will often be able to advise which preparation is the most effective as they will probably have been dispensing the drug to patients for years. Don't be shy to ask for their advice.

Chapter 13: Practical procedures

Even those with absolutely no hand–eye coordination can master practical procedures. Most importantly, practice makes perfect. Remember that mistakes are inevitable, so don't be too hard on yourself when you screw up – everyone does. Just be cautious at first and never be afraid to ask for help.

This section is aimed to guide you through most procedures you will encounter as an House Officer. You will no doubt soon develop your own tricks to perfect your performance.

General hints

• Always tell the patient what you are doing and why.
• Never do a procedure unless you have been supervised at least once.
• Order and space make procedures much easier. Before starting a procedure, get everything you need ready on a trolley. Make room for used sharps. Take a sharps bin to where you are working or have a kidney dish ready for sharps. Make sure you have enough local anaesthetic, needles and gloves.
• Consider taking the patient to a side room for the procedure, rather than performing it at the bedside which can be embarrassing for the patient and others on the ward.
• A warm, confident approach is most useful even if you are barrel of nerves

inside. It relaxes the patient and in turn will relax you.
• However, never be afraid to ask for help. It is really stupid to risk your reputation and the patient's well-being in order to prove bravado. People will trust you much more if they can rely on you to ask for help when necessary. In any case, seniors and nurses love showing off their skills.
• Always wear gloves. The most unlikely people have Hep B.
• Remember that you can ask nurses for help in positioning and reassuring the patient.
• Use local anaesthetic for all but the smallest procedures.
• Keep a vial of atropine and a syringe to hand for procedures that involve puncturing serosal linings (pleura, peritoneum), as vaso-vagal events are reasonably common. Give one ampoule (0.6 mg) IV stat if the patient feels faint.
• Remember that you always have more time than you think, even during emergency procedures. If necessary hand your bleep to a nursing or medical colleague while 'scrubbed up'. Less haste more speed is a good maxim for invasive procedures.

Arterial blood gases

Bleeding tendency is a relative contraindication for taking ABGs. Ask a senior for advice if you are in doubt about whether or not to proceed. Always apply pressure for at least 5 minutes after taking ABGs from patients on warfarin or heparin.

Arteries in order of preference:

1 Radial—check collateral blood supply from the ulnar artery (especially if there is a history of wrist trauma) by asking the patient to make a tight fist and applying pressure over the radial artery. Ask the patient to relax the hand. If it remains white after 10 seconds, try the other arm.

2 Femoral—the problem here is that it is easy to hit the vein by mistake. Also, you really need to apply strong pressure to the puncture site for at least 5 minutes after taking blood.

3 Brachial—use this as a last resort. Use a 20–22 G needle. The femoral is easier as it is much larger and less likely to thrombose.

Have ready

1 Lignocaine.
2 One 2 ml syringe.
3 One 23–25 G needle.

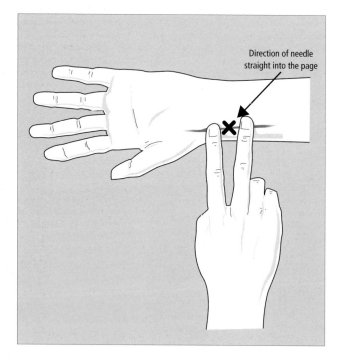

Fig. 13.1 Radial arterial puncture.

4 Heparin (1000 U/ml).
5 Povidone or iodine swabs or alchohol swabs.
6 Sterile swabs/cotton wool balls.
7 Syringe cap (keep a personal stock, not all wards have these). Many hospitals supply special heparinized syringes, e.g. 'Pulsator' for taking ABGs.
8 Plastic bag or carton with a few ice cubes at the bottom.

The procedure (see Figs 13.1 & 13.2)

1 Ask your colleagues where the blood gas machine is and how to read it before taking blood (it is often in ITU or A&E).
2 Draw up 0.5 ml of heparin into a 2 ml syringe, withdrawing the plunger fully to coat the syringe walls. Expel the heparin completely. You only need a few molecules to prevent the blood from clotting.

3 Wrist punctures are painful. It is a good idea to clean the skin and infiltrate superficially with a small bleb of local anaesthetic if there is no emergency.
4 Hold the syringe at a 60–90° angle to the skin and slowly advance the needle maintaining very slight negative pressure on the syringe. A flush of bright red blood indicates successful puncture. Keep very still and gently aspirate 1–2 ml.
5 Withdraw and apply pressure for at least 3 minutes (5 minutes if the patient is anticoagulated).
6 Expel all air from the syringe, tapping air bubbles towards the nozzle. Cap the syringe carefully and either take to the ABG machine immediately or place on ice and read as soon as possible (1 hour). Ice in a specimen bag is helpful to have ready so that you are not in such a panic to get to the ABG reading machine.

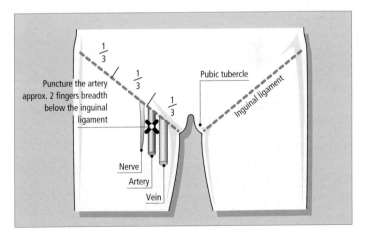

Fig. 13.2 Femoral arterial puncture.

If you fail

• Re-direct the needle without coming out of the skin. Try aiming the needle at a more shallow angle. This allows a steadier approach. Withdraw and try again.
• If you hit bone, withdraw while gently aspirating.

Hints

• It is important to expel all the air from the sample. Once this is done ice only serves to slow cellular use of O_2 which is negligible over 60 minutes.
• Don't expect immediate ABG changes after adjusting someone's O_2 supply. It takes up to 20 minutes for the ABGs to equilibrate to a change in inspired O_2 concentration. If a reading looks suspiciously high or low, repeat it.
• You can tell the difference between arterial and venous blood by its percentage saturation: 50% or less suggests venous blood, while 80% or above is certainly arterial.

Interpreting arterial blood gases

Normal ABG values are shown in Table 13.1.

Points to consider when interpreting arterial blood gases

For a full explanation of acid–base disorders consult any good medical textbook.

P_{O_2}

First ask yourself, does the patient have abnormally low O_2 for them? What is their baseline P_{O_2} value? Many patients with chronic respiratory disease live quite happily with a P_{O_2} of 7.5 kPa so don't get too flustered by an apparently terrible P_{O_2} value. Check the results of previous ABGs when the patient was well to see how much they have decompensated. (If you do not have previous results to hand you may need to seek senior advice on how to proceed.)

Next check if the patient is retaining CO_2. This will determine the amount of O_2 therapy you can give (see p. 72).

Remember that the O_2 saturation curve for Hb is a steep sigmoid curve that starts to plateau around a P_{O_2} of 9.1 kPa (70 mmHg). This means a patient may have a P_{O_2} of 8.5 kPa and still have better than 90% O_2 saturation. However, in the steep part of the curve (between P_{O_2} of 6–8 kPa), small changes in P_{O_2} dramatically affect O_2 saturation and are very clinically significant.

pH

Is it normal or is there an acidosis (pH < 7.35) or an alkalosis (pH > 7.45)? If either exists, decide if it is metabolic or

Table 13.1 Normal ABG values.

pH	7.35–7.45
P_{CO_2}	4.3–6.0 kPa
Base excess	+/– 2 mmol/l
P_{O_2}	10.5–14 kPa
Plasma HCO_3	22–26 mmol/l
O_2 saturation	95–100%

respiratory and whether or not it is compensated (see Table 13.2).

A compensated acid–base disorder suggests more chronic disease, over days to weeks, while an uncompensated acidosis or alkalosis suggests a more acute disorder. In general, the body compensates for changes in pH by altering the respiratory rate (e.g. in metabolic acidosis, CO_2 is 'blown off') and regulating renal excretion of HCO_3. Except in acute illness, most acid–base disorders are compensated to some extent.

Serum electrolytes (Na, Cl and HCO_3)

If the patient is acidotic you will need to calcuate the anion gap ($[Na + K] - [Cl + HCO_3]$) in order to refine the differential diagnosis. DKA, lactic acidosis, certain toxins and the acidosis associated with renal failure all cause increased production of unmeasured anions, resulting in an increased anion gap.

Hints

• Don't forget to note if the patient is on O_2, and how much, when interpreting ABGs.

• A patient with a mixed picture, or who is well compensated, may have a normal pH. Check all the parameters of the ABG analysis, not just the pH and Po_2.

• If the results of the ABG analysis are very poor, you may have sampled venous blood. This is likely if the percentage saturation is 50% or less. Percentage saturation of arterial blood is usually over 80%.

• Patients with decompensated organ failure (e.g. cirrhosis, CCF, respiratory

Table 13.2 Interpreting acid–base disorders.

	pH	Pco_2	HCO_3	K+
ACIDOSIS *Metabolic*				
Early	↓	Normal	↓	Usually ↑
Compensated	Normal	↓	↓	Normal or ↓
Respiratory				
Early	↓	↑	Normal or ↑	↑
Compensated	Normal	↑	↑↑	
ALKALOSIS *Metabolic*				
Early	↑	Normal	↑	↓
Compensated	↑	Normal	↑↑	↑
Respiratory				
Early	↑	↓	Normal or ↓	↓
Compensated	Normal	↓	↓↓	Normal or ↑

Reproduced from Zilva J.F., Pannall P.R., Mayne P. (1989). *Clinical Chemistry in Diagnosis and Treatment.* Lloyd-Luke (Medical Books) Ltd, London.

or renal insufficiency) may have developed acid–base and electrolyte disturbances over weeks. Do not be tempted to correct them in a day. Rather, try to get the patient a little better each day and review according to the time frame over which the patient's illness developed.

Respiratory disease and arterial blood gases interpretation

Type 1 respiratory failure (pink puffer):
• Pao_2 less than 8.0 kPa (60 mmHg).
• $Paco_2$ less than 6.0 kPa (45 mmHg).
If stable, their ABGs will reveal a compensated respiratory alkalosis.

Type 2 respiratory failure (blue bloater):
• Po_2 less than 8.0 kPa (60 mmHg).
• Pco_2 greater than 6.0 kPa (45 mmHg).
If stable, their ABGs will reveal a compensated respiratory acidosis.

Bladder catheterization

Ask an experienced colleague to supervise your first attempt and ensure that you know the procedure before your first night call. Female nurses usually catheterize women; you usually have to catheterize men.

Men

Have ready

1 Catheterization pack – contains kidney bowl, gauze swabs, sterile towels, etc.
2 Sterile gloves.
3 Cleaning solution.
4 Sterile tube of lignocaine jelly.
5 10 ml syringe and 10 ml sterile water.
6 Several Foley catheters. For the first attempt, 14 G is the usual size. Use a silastic catheter (which is firmer) for problematic catheterizations or when longer term catheterization is anticipated.
7 Urine bag and stand.

The procedure

1 Get a clean trolley which has been swabbed with an alcohol swipe and place the catheter pack on it. Also get a catheter stand.
2 Wash your hands thoroughly.
3 Wheel the trolley to the patient's bedside, draw the curtains and fully expose the patient's penis. Make sure there are no bedclothes in the way that might dirty the working area. UTIs are easy to induce with catherization.
4 Tell the patient what you are about to do and why you are doing it.
5 Without touching the sterile contents themselves, open the catheter pack, sterile gloves, tube of lignocaine jelly, syringe, water and catheter onto the catheter tray (or a sterile surface). Pour the cleaning solution (some hospitals use sterile saline alone) into a receptacle.
6 Put on gloves.
7 Drape the sterile towels or paper sheets to leave only the patient's penis exposed.
8 Gently retract the foreskin and clean the urethral opening with cleaning solution, keeping one hand clean for inserting the catheter.
9 Gently squeeze the contents of the tube of lignocaine jelly into the urethra, massaging the underside of the penis to work the jelly towards the bladder.

10 Open the catheter wrapping at the tip end only and insert the catheter into the urethra, withdrawing the plastic covering in stages as you go. This is the trickiest part of the procedure. Make sure the end is in the kidney bowl to collect urine. You should get some urine back when you reach the bladder from all but the most dehydrated patients.

11 If you feel resistance, gently pull the shaft of the penis upwards. In some cases pulling the penis down between the legs is more useful. *Never* use force.

12 Once fully inserted, inflate the catheter balloon with 5–10 ml of sterile water by placing the syringe directly over the proximal opening (no needle) and pushing hard. Stop immediately if the patient experiences pain as the balloon may be in the urethra. Once inflated, gently pull the catheter until you feel resistance of the balloon so that you are sure that it is stable in the bladder.

13 Gently pull back the foreskin. If you cannot, gently try again. If the foreskin genuinely gets stuck and starts to swell, get senior help immediately. Paraphimosis is a medical emergency.

14 Connect the end of the catheter to the bag and mount on a catheter stand.

15 Briefly document the procedure in the notes and record any significant volume of urine (>10–20 ml) that was collected in the kidney dish in the patient's fluid chart, particularly if the patient is in renal failure.

16 Send a sample of urine for MC&S.

If you fail

• The catheter may be blocked with jelly. Aspirate the catheter with the sy-ringe or gently massage the bladder above the pubic bone to encourage urine flow.

• The patient may have a large prostate or penile stricture. For strictures, a smaller size catheter should be used – proceed with care and be ready to abandon the procedure! For large prostates, *larger* catheters are useful, particularly stiff, silastic ones.

• If after several attempts with different size catheters you cannot access the bladder, never be shy of calling for help. Even the most senior urologists have trouble sometimes and can show you tricks for really difficult urethras.

• Supra-pubic catheterization is a useful last resort. Again, ensure supervision before attempting this alone as you risk perforating bowel.

Women

Have ready

Same equipment as for the men.

The procedure

1 Position the patient as for a vaginal examination. Ask her to lie flat on her back, knees bent, feet together and to allow her knees to fall down in full abduction.

2 Part the labia minora and clean the area with cleaning solution.

3 Locate the urethral opening just posterior to the clitoris and introduce a well lubricated catheter tip. Female catheterization is usually much less problematic than for males because they have no prostate and a really short urethra.

• As you will probably only be asked to

catheterize women that the experienced nurses cannot manage, get taught how to do this before you get called. Be aware of underlying causes for the problem such as tumours. If concerned, do a PV and do not be shy to call for help from a senior nurse.

Blood cultures

If you are going to the trouble of doing blood cultures it is better to do two sets from different sites, particularly if accurate diagnosis is very important. Three sets should be taken at 2–3 hourly intervals for suspected SBE.

Have ready

1 1 or 2 sets of culture bottles (some hospitals now use a single type of culture bottle for both aerobic and anaerobic cultures).
2 Two 20 ml syringes and needles.
3 Lots of alcohol swabs.

The procedure

1 Select a vein.
2 Clean the skin with alcohol, from the centre out. Allow to dry.
3 Without relocating the vein, cannulate and withdraw at least 10 ml of blood for each set of cultures.
4 Withdraw and inject at least 5 ml into each bottle.
5 Place in incubator as soon as possible.

Hints

• It is not necessary to change needles between taking blood and inserting it into the culture bottles. There is in-

creased risk of needlestick injury and little increase in contamination.
• It is also unnecessary to clean flip–cap culture-bottle tops.
• The above technique is fine for easy veins. If not, use a dressing pack, iodine, swabs, etc. and scrub up after you have got the patient ready. Keep your gloves sterile, as this will allow you to palpate for veins. You can also palpate for veins *through* an alcohol swab.

Blood letting

Have ready

1 Tourniquet.
2 Needles (green or blue).
3 Syringe(s) of adequate size for the bloods you need to take.
4 Alcohol swab(s).
5 Cotton wool ball or small plaster.
6 Blood tubes.
7 A sharps container.
• Vacutainers are much quicker to use than needles and syringes but have no 'flashback' to let you know when you have entered the vein. Therefore it is probably a good idea to use syringes and needles at first.

The procedure

1 Put on gloves.
2 Tell the patient what you are doing and why.
3 Choose the preferred arm (*not* a drip arm); tighten the tourniquet above the elbow and find a vein (see below). Visualize which way the needle will slide along the vein.
4 Swab the insertion area.
5 Put the needle on the syringe. Hold-

ing the patient's skin taut around the vein, gently but firmly advance the needle through the skin and subcutaneous fat into the vein. With practice you feel the vein give way when you are through. You should get a small 'flashback' in the base of the syringe.

6 Holding the syringe and needle in the arm very still, steadily draw back the syringe until you have enough blood.

7 Undo the tourniquet *before* withdrawing the needle.

8 Apply pressure to the puncture site with cotton wool or have the patient do so.

9 Taking care not to stick yourself, insert the needle into the blood tubes and allow the vacuum to withdraw the blood. (Some labs recommend that you remove the needle from the syringe, uncap the tube, and gently squirt the blood directly into the tube. This prevents needlestick injuries. In practice, very few House Officers we know use this technique.) Never squirt blood into the tube through small needles as this risks haemolysis and false readings.

10 Tidy up, especially sharps.

11 Send blood to the lab.

Choosing a vein

Ask the patient for his or her preferred arm. Usually the left arm is best for right-handed patients. Obvious forearm or cubital fossa veins are good. In dialysis patients, never use their AV fistula arm.

If you can't find a vein

1 Hang the arm over the edge of the bed, 'milking' it or tapping the back of the hand.

2 Use a sphygmomanometer; it is better than a tourniquet. Pump it up to diastolic pressure, asking the patient to pump their hand. For problematic patients use a sphygmomanometer first off.

3 Immerse the arm or hand in a bowl of warm water for 2 minutes; pump the sphygmomanometer up with the arm in the water; dry the arm and quickly look for veins.

4 Pump up the sphygmomanometer to above systolic pressure, asking the patient to exercise the hand until it aches (1–2 minutes), then release the pressure to diastolic level. The lactic acid produced as a result of anaerobic metabolism is a potent vasodilator. This method is painful. Use as a last resort.

Hints

• Always gently invert filled tubes containing anticoagulant so that no clotting occurs (e.g. haematology tubes).
• For the same reason, don't over-fill heparinized tubes – they will clot.
• Paediatric tubes, which only require a few drops of blood, can be used for patients with very difficult veins.
• Find out from the labs how much blood is really necessary for standard tests at your hospital. Often you need very little.
• Try removing the rubber stopper of the bottle if you need to put more blood in the bottle and you have lost the vacuum. Gently squirt blood from the syringe directly into the bottle having removed the needle (to avoid haemolysis).

Cannulation (Venflon/line insertion) (see Fig. 13.3)

No matter how much of a klutz you think you are, you will soon be inserting cannulae with the best of them. Practice really is the only way to be good at this. Here we outline the basic procedure with a trouble-shooting guide; the best way to learn the procedure is to get someone to show you.

Have ready

1 Tourniquet or sphygmomanometer.
2 Appropriate size cannula (see Table 13.3).
3 Cannula dressing (wing-shaped).
3 5–10 ml syringe.
4 Saline flush.
5 Alcohol swab(s).
6 Cotton wool ball/small plaster.
7 Bandage and tape.

The basic procedure

1 Put on gloves.
2 Tell the patient what you are doing and why.
3 Choose the preferred arm. Tighten the tourniquet above the elbow and find a vein (see below). Visualize which way

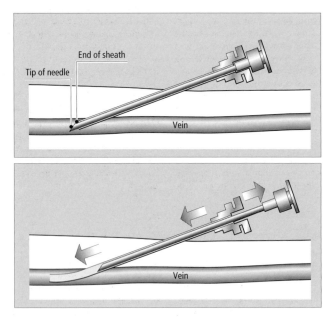

Fig. 13.3 Cannulating a vein.

Table 13.3 Cannulae sizes.

Colour	Size	Use
Blue	22 G	Small, fragile veins
Pink	20 G	IV drugs and fluid administration
Green	18 G	Blood transfusions, fluids
Yellow	17 G	As above
Grey	16 G	Rapid fluid administration, GI bleeds
Orange	14 G	Very rarely used, major bleeds

the needle will slide along the vein.

4 Swab the insertion area and allow the alcohol to dry (or it will sting).

5 Firmly advance the needle through the skin and subcutaneous fat into the vein. With practice you feel the vein give way when you are through. You should get a small 'flashback' of blood in the base of the cannula.

6 Holding the cannula in the arm very still, withdraw the metal stylet and *simultaneously* advance the plastic cannulae into the vein.

7 Undo the tourniquet and secure the cannula with a dressing. It is a good idea to secure the cannula with a covering bandage to prevent it catching on bed-clothes.

8 Tidy up, especially sharps.

Choosing a vein

1 Ask the patient for his or her preferred arm. Usually the left arm is best for right-handed patients. Remember that the dorsum of the hand is more convenient for you, but less so for the patient. Obvious forearm or cubital fossa veins are good (in dialysis patients, never use their AV fistula arm).

2 Avoid sites where two vein joins are tethered. While these can be easier to cannulate, the drip is more likely to tissue as a result of poor flexibility.

3 Avoid foot veins except as a last resort. They thrombose more readily and are prone to infection.

4 Avoid crossing joints.

5 Shave hairy arms for ease of cannulation and to reduce pain when removing the drip.

6 Palpate the vein, visualizing which way the needle will run along it.

If you can't find a vein, see p. 141 (blood letting).

Hints

• For squeamish patients Emla anaesthetic cream is extremely useful. Keep a tube handy. Apply over selected veins and cover with an occlusive dressing. Simply wipe off in 30 minutes to 1 hour and site the drip as usual. Injection of local anaesthetic is less useful as it often obscures the vein.

• It is helpful to take blood at the same time as putting in the cannula. This must not be done with 'precious' veins. Once the cannula is secured, elevate the arm above the level of the left atrium. Remove the cap and place a syringe into the back of the cannula. Lower the arm (sometimes you need to reinflate the cuff gently) and very gently aspirate the required amount of blood.

• Pink, rather than green cannulae, are adequate for most routine purposes, such as saline infusions or IV drugs.

Saving a dying drip or cannula

When asked to re-site a cannula because it has tissued:

1 Ask whether or not it is still really necessary.

2 Many lines can be flushed gently with 5 ml of heparinized saline that clears any minor blockage. Small syringes (2 ml) are most effective at clearing minor blocks.

3 Always remove the cannula if the site is inflamed.

Times when a cannula MUST be in place, even at night

• The acutely ill or unstable patient.
• Hypovolaemia or poor oral intake.
• Serious danger of blood or fluid loss.
• Certain IV drug infusions – antibiotics, cardiac infusions, heparin, etc.

Central lines

Ensure that you are supervised for your first attempts; this procedure has the potential for some big time complications. The two most commonly used

veins are the internal jugular and subclavian, usually on the right side. Other under-used approaches include the femoral vein and the median basilic vein, both of which are technically easier but don't last as long. The same principles apply to all CVP lines.

Indications for CVP lines

• Measurement of CVP.
• Infusing certain drugs and TPN.
• Inserting Swan-Ganz catheters or pacing wires.

Insertion of central lines

When to use the jugular approach

1 Clotting problems, typically when the INR is greater than 5 or the platelet count is less than $100 \times 10^9/l$.

2 Respiratory disease where a pneumothorax might be life threatening although they can still occur with this approach.

Have ready

1 Central line set.
2 Standard dressing pack.
3 Betadine.
4 Sterile gown and gloves.
5 One large sterile drape.
6 10 ml 1% lignocaine.
7 Two 10 ml syringes.
8 Heparinized saline (Hepsal) to flush lines.
9 25 G (orange) and 21 G (green) needles.
10 Suturing material (2-0 or 3-0 silk or prolene).
11 Scalpel blade.

12 Two adhesive dressings.
13 500 ml bag of saline and giving set.
14 CVP manometer.

The procedure (see Fig. 13.4)

1 Have trolley ready (sterile contents laid out). Remove all pillows. Tilt the bed to lower the patient's head (to fill the neck veins). Tell the patient what you are about to do and why. Reassure them that while it is uncomfortable to lie still and backwards for about 20 minutes, that the procedure is not painful.

2 Wash your hands well and put on gloves.

3 Flush the giving set and CVP manometer with heparin saline.

4 Clean a wide area of skin from the inside out around the puncture site and cover with the drape.

5 Flush the central venous cannula and connecting tubing with saline.

6 Check that the guidewire passes

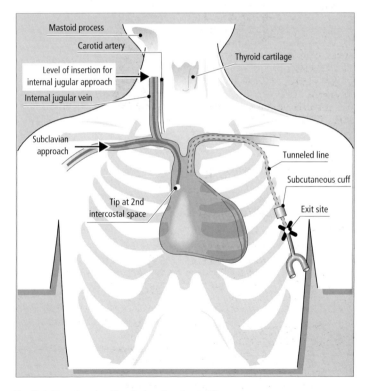

Fig. 13.4 Illustration of positions for insertion of central lines.

through the large bore needle and determine which is the soft, 'vessel-friendly' end.

Cannulating the right internal jugular vein

1 Feel for the pulse of the carotid artery with the left hand. With the right hand, infiltrate local anaesthetic subcutaneously at the level of the thyroid cartilage and lateral to the carotid artery.
2 Whilst guarding the carotid artery with the left hand, insert a green needle attached to a 10 ml syringe, at an angle of 45° to the neck, heading towards the right anterior superior iliac spine. The right nipple in males is also a good landmark.
3 Advance slowly, aspirating for blood. The vein is superficial. Do not go more than a few centimetres. If you fail to get blood, withdraw slowly, you may have gone through the vein. If this doesn't work, try again, slightly more medially. If by mistake you do hit the carotid artery don't panic; apply strong pressure for 5 minutes.
4 When you have found the vein, withdraw the needle. Take the large bore needle with attached syringe and follow the line taken with the green needle.

Cannulating the subclavian vein

1 Visualize the sternoclavicular and acromioclavicular joints to find the intersection of the medial one-third and lateral two-thirds of the clavicle.
2 Beginning about 1 cm below the clavicle, infiltrate local anaesthetic right up to the clavicle, including the peri-

osteum, using a blue needle.
3 Insert a green needle through the anaesthetized area and advance towards the clavicle, aiming for the suprasternal notch (see Fig. 13.4). Aspirate and infiltrate with local anaesthetic as you go. Once you reach the clavicle, work your way down it until the needle goes just under the inferior surface. You usually will not reach the vein with a green needle.
4 Repeat step 3 with the large bore needle, aspirating as you go. If you fail, aim slightly more upwards.

Inserting the guidewire

1 Before inserting the guidewire, ensure that you can aspirate blood freely through the needle.
2 Ask the patient to breathe out. As s/he is doing so, remove the syringe and place your thumb over the lumen to prevent air entry.
3 Insert the soft end of the guidewire. It should pass with minimal resistance. *Never* force it. If it won't pass, check you can still aspirate blood and try again. If it still won't pass, change the angle of the needle slightly.
4 Pass about 50% of the length of the wire and remove the needle, holding the end of the wire firmly.
5 Nick the skin at the line's entry point with a scalpel blade. Thread the dilator and twist it down over the wire to the hilt. Remove the dilator, taking care not to pull out the wire, then thread the catheter. Remove the wire.
6 Check you can aspirate blood from each lumen of the catheter. Flush with heparinized saline (Hepsal) before clamping each lumen.

7 Secure with two sutures and place two occlusive clear dressings like a sandwich over the cannula.

8 Do a CXR to check the line's position and to exclude a pneumothorax.

Hints

• For the subclavian approach, placing a 1 l bag of saline between the patient's shoulder blades makes access easier.

• The breathless patient need only be flat or head down for cannulation of the vein and insertion of the guidewire. The rest can be done sitting up.

• Always take the pulse following the procedure. Frequent ectopics suggest the catheter is in the right ventricle and should be pulled back into the vein.

• If you hit the carotid or subclavian artery apply firm pressure for a full 5 minutes.

• Never attempt both subclavian veins without obtaining a CXR.

Problems with temporary and tunneled central lines

You will often be called to sort out line problems. The commonest are:

Sepsis. If a patient with a central line develops a fever, take peripheral and central blood cultures. If the patient is clearly septic (temperature >38 °C, tachycardia, pain/inflammation around entry site) discuss removing the line with your senior. Tunneled lines can sometimes be treated with antibiotics if the patient is otherwise well, but this cannot be done for short term lines when the track is much shorter. After removal of any central line, always cut

the tip off with a sterile pair of scissors and send it for culture.

Blocked lumen. This is prevented by daily flushing with heparinized saline (available on most wards in prepared vials). If the line is blocked, flush using a 1–2 ml syringe with heparinized saline, applying moderate pressure. Remember to put in a heparin–saline lock after flushing. Lines near the lumen sometimes wind around on themselves; simple unwinding can sometimes alleviate apparently severe blocks. If still no luck, a dilute solution of urokinase can be instilled by repeated aspiration and injection. Leave it for 30 minutes after which you can try flushing again.

Hints

• Taking blood from central lines should only be performed as a last resort. You need to discard the first 15 ml of blood and use a good aseptic technique. Do not take samples for aminoglycoside levels from a central line as these drugs are adsorbed by the cannula.

• A 1–2 ml syringe is more effective for unblocking cannulae than a 5 or 10 ml syringe.

Using central lines

Hickman and Groschong lines are tunneled lines intended for long-term use such as for chemotherapy or TPN. Groschong lines have a special two-way valve system at the tip of each lumen that prevents blockage after flushing and facilitates taking of blood samples. However, the valve excludes the use of the line for CVP measurements. It is extremely useful to know how to handle these lines. Infection is the major problem and most patients are trained in looking after their own line. They are very critical of sloppy technique. Therefore, before handling a line, ask a nurse or medical colleague to give you a quick tutorial. The basic technique outlined below is a guide only. Different units use different IV connectors, bungs, etc. For setting up an IV, giving drugs or taking blood via a tunneled line you will need to:

1 Open up:
  • Dressing pack.
  • Sterile gloves.

Fig. 13.5 Diagrammatic illustration of CVP reading.

- One 5 ml syringe and heparin–saline or saline.
- One sterile bung (end plug for cannula).
- Four alcohol swabs.
- Cleaning solution, e.g. betadine solution, and container.

2 Get an assistant (always handy).

3 Scrub up.

4 Keep one hand absolutely sterile.

5 Handle the line with dry sterile gauze.

6 Remove the bung from the end of the line using a swab and discard.

7 Always open and shut the gate or clamp between procedures.

8 Attach drip or take bloods as appropriate.

Measuring the CVP
(see Fig. 13.5)

The CVP is measured with reference to a fixed point, either the mid-axillary line or the manubriosternal angle. The pressures at the manubriosternal angle will be about 5–7 cm lower than those at the mid-axillary line. It does not matter which you use, as long as you remain consistent.

1 Lie the patient flat. Adjust the scale so that the 10 cm mark is opposite the chosen reference point (marked with an indelible pen). If you use the true '0 cm' level you cannot measure negative values.

2 A three-way tap controls the flow of fluid between the IV bag, the CVP reading scale and the patient. Adjust the tap to run fluid from the bag up to the 30 cm mark on the manometer. Set the tap to connect the patient to the manometer. The manometer fluid level should swing with respiration and settle. The CVP is measured in cm of water.

Hints

1 Learn to measure the CVP yourself and take the time to ensure that nursing staff are familiar with doing CVP measurements. It is easy to get it wrong.

2 Normal values for CVP:

Using the 10 cm mark aligned with the manubriosternal angle: 7–14 cm.

Using the 10 cm mark aligned with the mid-axillary line: 11–18 cm.

(Subtract 10 cm if using the true 0 cm mark.)

3 The CVP reading should be regarded with suspicion if right atrial pressure is likely to be abnormal:

- Raised intrathoracic pressure (tension pneumothorax).
- Altered intravascular volume (fluid overload or hypovolaemia).
- Abnormal venous tone (NB catecholamine release can maintain CVP readings despite significant blood loss). Other drugs can cause dramatic loss of tone and drops in CVP.
- Abnormal right ventricular function: CCF, pericardial tamponade/constriction, acute RVF. The CVP may be markedly raised following right-sided AMI or large PE. The CVP in these situations is an unreliable guide to fluid status. If called to see a patient with a rising or falling CVP think of the above approach to guide you.

Chest drains

You are unlikely to be expected to insert a chest drain, but you will be expected to manage and remove chest drains. The decision to remove a drain should be taken by your seniors. The following paragraphs give some general guidelines to maintaining and removing drains (see Fig. 13.6).

Indications

Pneumothorax.
Haemothorax or empyema.
Large pleural effusion.

Managing a chest drain

Pneumothorax

1 Check for an air leak by asking the patient to cough. A bubbling drain implies an air leak from an unsealed hole, fistula or a leak in the tubing. You may need to apply suction to the drain if you suspect a hole or fistula.
2 After the lung has re-expanded and the drain is no longer bubbling, clamp and re-X-ray. If there is no pneumothorax and the fluid is cleared, the drain can be removed.

Effusion/haemothorax

1 Large effusions can drain over several days, up to a maximum of 1 litre/hour and not more than 4 litres/day (otherwise there is a risk of 'reflex' pulmonary oedema). Remove the drain when the CXR reveals no further fluid.

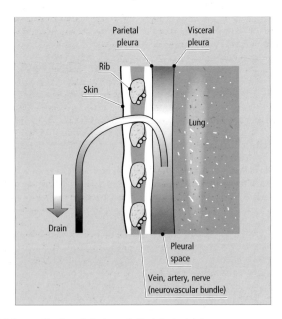

Fig. 13.6 Cross section through chest cage to illustrate chest drain.

2 For recurrent effusions you may consider chemical pleurodesis; discuss with your team.

3 Empyema drains require special consideration. Get a specialist opinion.

How to remove a drain

Have ready

1 Gloves.
2 Clamping forceps.
3 Pair of scissors.
4 One occlusive dressing.

The procedure

1 Clamp the tube with the forceps.

2 The entry point of the tube should have been secured with a purse-string suture that must be untied (not cut) and the ends firmly pulled to seal the hole as the tube slides out. Take your time the first few times you do this. It is easy to lose the stitching.

3 Withdraw the tube with positive intra-thoracic pressure by asking the patient to blow hard against a closed nose and mouth ('Make your ears pop'). You should hear the hiss of the expulsion of the last bit of air as the end comes out. Quickly pull the purse string to seal the hole. Apply an occlusive dressing.

4 Do a CXR to assess the success of the drain and as a comparison for future X-rays.

Hint

• Have a 4×4 cm gauze swab to hand to place over the hole in the event of a failed purse-string closure. Later, replace this with a large clear occlusive dressing over the hole.

Electrocardiogram

Many indications, especially history of IHD; DM; hypertension; SOB; chest pain; swollen leg; pre-op. ECGs don't take much time and are harmless; if in doubt, just do one.

The procedure

1 Have the patient lie with their chest exposed. Explain to them what you are doing and reassure them that there is no way that they will get an electric shock.

2 Attach limb leads to the inner aspect of the forearm just below the wrist and the outer aspects of the leg above the ankle. The wires are usually labelled but if not the colour code is most often as follows:

Red = right arm
Yellow = left arm
Green = left leg
Black = right leg

3 Ensure good contact with electrode jelly (you can also use KY jelly).

4 For chest leads see Fig. 13.7.

Hints

• Doing ECGs is mostly a hassle when you don't know where to find a portable ECG machine. To save sleep, make sure you know where one is before you go to bed, as well as where you can find replacement paper, electrode jelly or disposable electrode pads for the lucky few hospitals that have them.

Preventing spurious results:

• The patient should be completely relaxed. Explain that the procedure is completely painless and harmless.

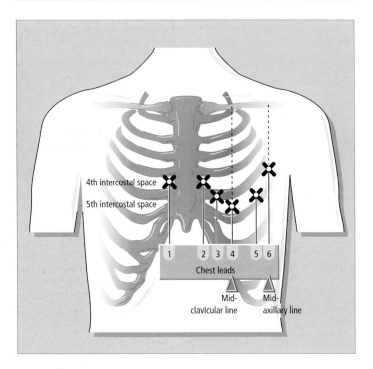

Fig. 13.7 ECG chest lead placement.

• Make sure the chest lead electrodes do not overlap.

• Lightly shave very hairy areas for proper contact.

• If the patient has a hand tremor (e.g. Parkinsons) attach the leads higher up the arm.

• The black (right leg) lead is an earth lead and can be attached to any part of the body. It has no bearing on the result.

• For leg amputees, the green (left leg) lead can be placed on either leg. However, the arm leads must not be crossed. For an arm amputee, ensure that the arm electrodes are equidistant from the heart (they may be placed on the shoulders).

Reading ECGs (see pp. 48–51)

Exercise stress test

Exercise (ECG) stress tests take approximately 20 minutes to perform. Your job is to encourage the patient to attain their peak heart rate if possible (= 220 − patient age), and to watch their ECG closely. Your aim is to detect and measure the severity of coronary artery disease, and to uncover arrhythmias.

Relative contraindications (discuss with senior)

Aortic stenosis.
Hypertrophic obstructive cardiomyopathy.
LBBB on ECG.
Systolic BP > 200 mmHg; diastolic BP > 100 mmHg.
Unstable angina.
Uncontrolled arrhythmias.
Note: Beta-blockers should be stopped 2 days before the test.

The procedure

1 Make sure that there is resuscitation equipment immediately available. Approximately 1 per 4000 patients arrests during stress tests. Also have GTN ready.
2 Assess peak heart rate = 220 − patient age.
3 Follow the instructions of the ECG technician, who has followed the protocol many times.
4 *Stop the test* if the patient complains of:
  • Increasingly severe chest pain or other symptoms (such as faintness or dyspnoea). Consider administering GTN.
  • A fall in systolic BP of more than 20 mmHg.
  • A fall in heart rate.
  • VT or VF.
  • Progressive ST elevation.
  • ST depression greater than or equal to 2 mm.
  • Three or more consecutive ventricular ectopics.
  • Peak heart rate is attained.

5 You must remain present at all times and monitor BP and pulse at regular intervals (ask the technician for local protocol). This includes the recovery period when the test may become positive, or (horrors) the patient may go into VT. (Be ready to resuscitate.)

Glucose tolerance test

Indications

Suspected diabetes mellitus.

Have ready

1 The patient should have fasted overnight.
2 75 g oral glucose dissolved in a glass of water.
3 Apparatus for taking blood with grey (glucose) tube.

The procedure

1 Take a fasting sample for blood glucose in a grey tube.
2 Give the patient the oral glucose with the water to drink over less than 5 minutes.
3 Take a second blood glucose sample after 2 hours.

Interpreting the results

1 Normal result: 2-hour glucose level is less than 7.8 mmol.
2 Impaired glucose tolerance: fasting plasma level less than 7.8 mmol and the 2-hour level between 7.8 and 11.1 mmol.
3 Diabetes confirmed: fasting plasma level greater than 7.8 mmol and the 2-hour level greater than 11.1 mmol.

Injections

Subcutaneous

Have ready

1 23–25 G needle.
2 Alcohol swab.

The procedure

1 Choose a fatty site and use the small-est possible needle.
2 Clean site with an alcohol swab and allow to dry.

3 Gently pinch a wad of skin and fat between your thumb and index finger.
4 Place the needle on the skin for 3 seconds at an angle of about 60° before pushing through the skin. This reduces the sensation of pain. Release the skin.
5 Aspirate to ensure you do not inject into a blood vessel.
6 Slowly depress the plunger. Rapid injection will cause pain.
If you aspirate blood, remove and replace the needle and explain to the patient the need to repeat the injection.

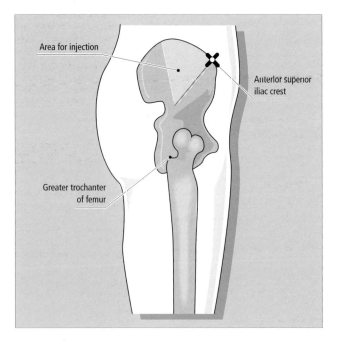

Fig. 13.8 Site for intramuscular injections.

Intramuscular

Have ready

As for SC.

The procedure

1 The deltoid muscle is usually good for small injections. If the patient is thin or wasted use the gluteal muscles — choose the upper and outer quadrant below the iliac crest to avoid the sciatic nerve by drawing an imaginary line between the anterior superior iliac spine and the greater trochanter of the femur, and injecting posteriorly to and above this line (see Fig. 13.8).
2 Pull the skin taut and inject at 90° to the skin (pulling the skin ensures that the injection doesn't leak after you pull the needle out).
3 Aspirate to ensure you do not inject into a blood vessel. Inject slowly.

Intercostal block

Indications

Very effective for severe, localized, pleuritic chest pain (e.g. localized pleuritis, metastases, fractured ribs). Intercostal blocks usually abolish pain and surprisingly the relief lasts longer than the action of the anaesthetic.

Have ready

1 Dressing pack and sterile gloves.
2 Betadine.
3 One 10 ml syringe.
4 One 23 G needle.
5 One 21 G needle.

6 5–10 ml 2% lignocaine or 0.5% bupivacaine (preferred, because it is longer acting).

The procedure

1 Identify the interspace(s) where the pain is arising and the spaces above and below. Prepare the skin in the mid-axillary line. Anaesthetize the skin using a 23 G needle just below the inferior margin of the rib with lignocaine. You need to deliver the drug close to the nerve.
2 Change needle to 21 G (green). Going through the same puncture site, advance at an upward angle again towards the inferior margin of the rib. The nerve lies inferiorly in the groove. If you hit bone, withdraw slightly and try again, slightly more inferiorly. Aspirate to ensure the needle is not in a vessel and slowly inject 1–2 ml of bupivacaine.
3 Repeat the procedure for the interspaces above and below.

Joint aspiration/injection

This is useful procedure to learn from an expert, especially if you are an aspiring GP. Superb aseptic technique is vital as is a sound knowledge of the anatomy. Each joint requires a slightly different approach but the basic technique is the same.

Aspiration

Indications

Diagnostic:
• Recent onset arthritis.

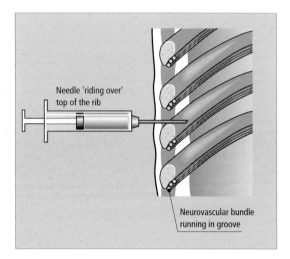

Fig. 13.9 Pleural aspiration (diagram shows an oblique section).

- To rule out infection (acute and chronic).
- Joint effusion.

Therapeutic:
  - Steroid injections.
  - Drainage of septic arthritis.

Have ready

1 Three syringes (5, 10 and 50 ml).
2 Two needles (25 G and 21 G).
3 Lignocaine 2%.
4 Sterile gloves.
5 Sterile dressing pack.
6 Betadine solution.
7 Three specimen containers and a fluoride tube (grey top) for infections.

The procedure

1 Written consent is advisable.

2 Find the site of maximal effusion and mark this point with indelible ink.
3 Scrub up and clean the area with betadine. Allow it to dry and wipe over the site of aspiration with an alcohol swab. Allow it to dry completely. Even small amounts of betadine will ruin your culture results.
4 Anaesthetize the area being careful to avoid injecting local anaesthetic into the joint – lignocaine is also bactericidal so will mess up cultures.
5 Insert the aspiration needle and advance it slowly whilst maintaining slight negative pressure. When you hit the effusion, tap it completely.
6 Never inject steroids if joint infection is a possibility. To inject steroids after tapping an effusion, disconnect the syringe leaving the needle in place. Attach the syringe containing the ster-

oid. Aspirate to ensure you are not in a vessel, then inject. There should be minimal resistance. Stop if you feel you are in the tissues and try again.

7 Remove the needle and apply pressure for a minute. Dress the wound.

Hints

• Phone microbiology to request urgent microscopy on the joint fluid. Some labs insist on special transport media when certain infections are suspected – get advice from the microbiologist.

• The sub-talar joint (below the ankle joint) is notoriously difficult to aspirate – get expert help.

Injecting joints

Many rheumatology departments teach a simple no-touch technique. The risk of infection following this method is no worse than that outlined above.

Have ready

1 Two 5 ml syringes – one for lignocaine (to anaesthetize the skin) if deemed necessary, and one for the steroid, +/– lignocaine.
2 Two alcohol swabs.
3 A small plaster.
4 Triamcinolone (5–20 mg) or methylprednisolone (10–40 mg) for steroid injections. The dose will depend on the size of the joint.

The procedure

1 Inform the patient of the small risk of infection (see above).
2 Draw up the lignocaine (if required) and the steroid for injection. The latter

is now available with lignocaine added. This limits the potentially painful response to the injection and lasts about 2–3 hours. Note that the lignocaine for skin anaesthesia is still advisable for squeamish patients.

3 Locate the site for injection; clean with an alcohol swab and allow to dry. Without touching the site again push through the skin and anaesthetize the skin down to the joint. Remember to aspirate to ensure you are not in a vessel. Remove and allow a minute for the local anaesthetic to work.

4 Repeat (3) except this time inject the joint with steroid. There should be minimal resistance to the injection.

5 Remove the needle and apply pressure for a minute. Dress the wound.

Hints

• Tell the patient that mild pain and redness can occur after steroid injections and may persist up to 24 hours. They are due to a reaction to the crystalline suspension used in long acting steroids, but be wary of iatrogenic infection.

• Never inject steroids if joint infection is a possibility.

Local anaesthesia (for any procedure)

Have ready

1 21 G and 23 G needle.
2 5–10 ml syringe.
3 Alcohol swabs.
4 1–2% lignocaine ampoules.

The procedure

1 Start with a 23–25 G needle. Infiltrate the skin and SC tissues raising a small bleb. If deeper anaesthesia is required, switch to a larger needle (21 G), wait 1 minute, then pass through the same puncture site.
2 Aspirate for blood before injecting anything. If you hit blood, withdraw a little and try again.
3 Wait at least 2 minutes for effect.

Hints

• Lignocaine lasts approximately 2 hours. Marcaine and bupivacaine are longer acting (8 hours) and useful for intercostal blocks.
• Use lignocaine with adrenaline for very vascular sites where you need to incise skin, as adrenaline causes vasoconstriction. *Never* use adrenaline for a nerve block of an extremity, e.g. a finger ring block.
• To work out the dose of lignocaine in mg/ml, multiply the percentage concentration by 10. Maximum dose of lignocaine within 24 hours:
   Without adrenaline: 3 mg/kg
   With adrenaline: 7 mg/kg

Lumbar puncture

Lumbar punctures are actually pretty easy once you get the hang of them. The thing to do is to reassure the patient that it is an uncomfortable but relatively painless procedure, and that it might take up to 30 minutes—so you don't feel rushed. Of all procedures, this one requires a slow, methodical approach for success.

Indications

Diagnostic:
• Meningitis, SAH, rarities.
Therapeutic:
• Intra-thecal drugs (never to be given by House Officers—a job for SHOs and above).

Contraindications (get help)

1 Local sepsis.
2 Raised ICP (vomiting, bradycardia, drowsiness, papilloedema).
3 Suspicion of a cord or posterior fossa mass.
4 Coagulopathy or platelet count <40.
• If patient is drowsy, unconscious or has evidence of raised ICP, request an urgent CT scan before doing an LP.

Have ready

1 LP pack or if none available:
2 Two sterile drapes.
3 One gallipot.
4 One pack gauze swabs.
5 One pack of cotton wool balls.
6 Two LP needles (an 18 G (yellow) or a 20 G (black); open one).
7 One sterile, disposable manometer.
8 Three sterile, 20 ml specimen containers.
9 Antiseptic (povidone/betadine solution or equivalent).
10 5–10 ml lignocaine 2%.
11 10 ml syringe.
12 23 G and 21 G needles.
13 Sterile gloves.

The procedure (see Fig. 13.10)

1 Obtain oral consent. Explain to the patient what you are doing, that the pro-

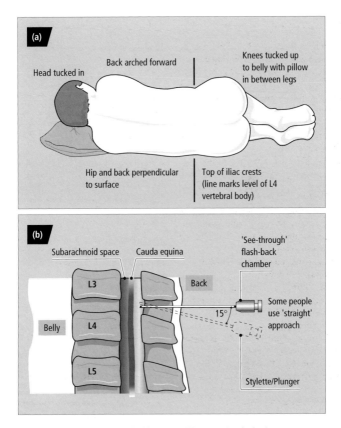

Fig. 13.10 (a) Patient position for lumbar puncture. (b) Approaches for lumbar puncture.

cedure may take some time but is not very painful – just uncomfortable.

2 Ask the patient to lie as indicated in Fig. 13.10 – with knees tucked up under the chin as much as possible (to draw the spinal cord out of the way of the needle). Ensure the vertebral column is parallel to the bed (the hips are exactly perpendicular to the edge of the bed).

3 Get an LP pack ready on a trolley with plenty of room to manoeuvre. Make room for sharps and dirty items.

4 Scrub up as for a sterile technique.

5 Prepare skin with betadine and cover with a sterile drape.

6 Unscrew the tops of the three sterile sample containers.

7 Locate the puncture site L3–L4 or

L4–L5 by drawing two imaginary lines, one joining the top of the iliac crests and the other running down the spine. These intersect at L3–L4. The spinal cord ends at L1–L2, so the L2–L3 interspace is safe if you cannot use the lower interspaces for some reason, but ensure the patient is properly curled up.

8 Anaesthetize using a 23 G needle for superficial skin and SC infiltration. Switch to a 21 G needle for deeper infiltration into the interspinous ligament. Inject slowly waiting at least 2 minutes for effect.

9 Assemble the LP equipment, check that the stylette moves freely within the needle, and check how to use the manometer taps.

10 Insert the needle in the midline between the two spinous processes. Advance towards the patient's umbilicus (slightly towards the head). Resistance increases as the needle passes through the interspinous ligament. A small 'give' is felt as the needle punctures the ligamentum flavum. Withdraw the stylette to check for a flash back of CSF. If there is no CSF, advance the needle a few millimetres and check again.

11 Attach the manometer, allow the patient to relax and measure the pressure (recorded in cm H_2O; normal range 6–15 cm). The level will fluctuate with respiration.

12 Disconnect the manometer. From the open end of the needle collect:
- 2–5 drops for biochemistry.
- 5–10 drops for bacteriology.
- Up to 5–10 drops for cytology.

13 Withdraw the needle slowly, taking care not to spill too many drops of CSF (causing a severe headache afterwards). Dress the wound.

14 The patient should lie flat for 4 hours. They may have a moderate headache afterwards. If they experience a severe headache they should inform the nurses or doctors.

If you fail

- Correct positioning is the key to success. If you fail, re-check the patient's position. Try another interspace if necessary.
- If the patient is anatomically 'difficult' (e.g. very large or has an abnormal spinal column), ask a more experienced senior or enlist the help of a radiologist who can do the LP under X-ray screening.
- You feel you are in the right place but no CSF – lightly rotate the needle through 90°; the bevel may be lying against a nerve root.

Hints

- Sedate the patient if required: 2.5–5 mg diazepam orally 30 minutes before the procedure. The patient needs to remain horizontal for at least 4 hours post-LP to reduce the incidence of severe headache. Warn the patient that headaches can occur up to 3 days after an LP.
- *Never* apply suction to a CSF needle.
- Subarachnoid haemorrhage is easily distinguishable from a bloody tap by uniform blood staining of the three consecutive samples and xanthochromia in the supernatant. The samples from a bloody tap gradually clear. Send samples for a cell count.

Mantoux test

Indication

A Mantoux tests for a delayed-type hypersensitivity reaction to a partially purified protein derivative from *Mycobacterium tuberculosis*. For routine pre-BCG skin testing the 10 unit dose of tuberculin PPO is used.

Have ready

1 Order PPD from pharmacy.
2 1 ml diabetic syringe (26 G 1 cm needle).
3 Alcohol swab.

The procedure

1 Dilute PPD to a concentration of 100 TU/ml.
2 Draw up 0.1 ml (10 TU) into a diabetic syringe.
3 Clean a small area on the left forearm (convention).
4 Indicate the area to be injected with a marker pen.
5 Keeping the needle almost horizontal to the skin, carefully insert the needle intra-dermally and inject 0.1 ml so that a small bleb is raised.
6 A negative reaction at 48 hours indicates a negative response.
7 Read at 72 hours. Measure the diameter of induration, not the erythema:
   • >10 mm = positive; suggestive of previous or current infection, not necessarily disease.
   • >20 mm = strongly positive, highly suggestive of active disease.

Nasogastric tubes

Nurses are usually experienced at inserting NG tubes; you are usually called only if they fail. Therefore it is a good idea to do a few before such a call. They are usually straightforward.

Have ready

1 An apron and non-sterile gloves.
2 Fresh NG tube – size 10 (small) to 16 (large).
3 Kidney bowl and catheter drainage bag.
4 KY jelly.
5 Glass of water.

The procedure

1 Sit the patient upright with chin on chest.
2 Tell the patient what you are doing and ask for their help in swallowing the tube.
3 Lubricate the tube with jelly and insert into a nostril. Gently advance the tube towards the occiput (not upwards). Ask the patient to swallow when they feel the tube at the back of their throat and advance the tube as they swallow. They may find swallowing the water simultaneously to be helpful.
4 To assess position: aspirate some contents using a small syringe and test with blue litmus paper to check the contents are gastric (blue litmus paper turns red on contact with acidic gastric juices); or, with a syringe, blow air down the tube whilst listening with a stethoscope over the stomach.
5 Attach the drainage bag.

If you fail

• Try the other nostril.
• Try oral insertion—ask the patient to swallow the tube.
• Sometimes NG tubes have two lumens. If you don't block off one lumen when syringing air through the other to check the position of the NG tube, it will appear (falsely) as if the tube is not in the stomach.
• Get help from a senior.
• Consider endoscopic placement under mild sedation.

Hints

• NG tubes are uncomfortable and predispose to sinusitis. Remove as soon as possible.
• Use fine-bore tubes for enteral feeding.

Peritoneal tap (paracentesis)

Like pleural aspiration paracentesis is remarkably straightforward and even quite fun. The procedure is identical to pleural aspiration except for the position of the patient and puncture site.

The procedure

1 Ask the patient to empty their bladder. Explain what you are doing and why. Stress that the procedure is painless except for initial anaesthesia.
2 Lie the patient as flat as possible.
3 Percuss out the ascites.
4 Scrub up, prepare the skin and drape.

Give local anaesthetic in the sites indicated in Fig. 13.11.
5 Follow the same procedure as for pleural aspiration (see below).
6 For therapeutic taps use a suprapubic or peritoneal dialysis catheter. These are usually supplied with drainage bags.
7 Send samples for biochemistry (protein, glucose, LDH), bacteriology (MC&S, ZN stain and TB culture) and cytology.

Hints

• Do not remove more than 500 ml in the first 10 minutes and no more than 1200 ml in 24 hours. More fluids risks hypotension but may be appropriate for some patients; check with your senior.
• Avoid going too close to old surgical scars as bowel may be attached to the abdominal wall.
• You may need to reposition the catheter or 'jiggle' the patient to maintain the flow.
• Bizarre cells on cytology often represent reactive mesothelial cells, not malignancy. Always get a formal report before embarking on a hunt for a tumour.
• Complications are rare but include perforated bowel, peritonitis, intra-abdominal haemorrhage and perforated bladder.
• Paracentesis is essential to rule out peritonitis in patients with cirrhosis and long standing ascites who become decompensated.

Pleural aspiration

Pleural aspiration is straightforward, although the idea of plunging tubing into

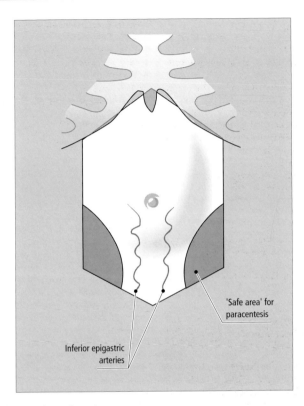

Fig. 13.11 Site for tapping ascites.

someone's chest sounds daunting. Ask a senior nurse or medical colleague to supervise your first one.

Indications

Diagnostic
• Infection.
• Malignancy.
Therapeutic
• Large effusions for relief of SOB.

Have ready

1 Dressing pack (some hospitals have a prepared pleural aspiration pack).
2 Sterile gloves.
3 One 10 ml syringe.
4 One green needle.
5 One blue needle.
6 10 ml 2% lignocaine.
7 Three specimen jars (sterile).
For therapeutic taps add:

8 One large bore IV cannula (brown or grey Venflon).

9 One three-way tap.

10 IV giving set and an empty, sterile bowl or saline bag.

The procedure

1 Confirm the size and extent of the effusion on the most recent CXR. Scrub up. Tell the patient what you are doing and how long it will take.

2 Sit the patient upright in bed or sit them on a stool leaning slightly forward over the side of the bed, resting their elbows on a pillow.

3 Select the insertion site by tapping out the effusion. The best sites are usually two to three spaces below the lowest point (angle) of the scapula or at the same level in the posterior axillary line. Avoid the mid-clavicular line on the left (the heart!).

4 Scrub up and drape as for a sterile procedure. Ensure you have a sterile, flat surface on which to put things.

5 Anaesthetize the skin first with a 23 G (blue) needle for superficial infiltration and then again with an 18 G (yellow) needle for deeper infiltration. The track of the needle should hug the upper border of the rib to avoid the neurovascular bundle (see Fig. 13.9). Always withdraw before injecting local anaesthetic to make sure you are not in a blood vessel. In the average person, you should aspirate pleural fluid at the full depth of a green needle.

6 Attach a 20 ml syringe to the end of a green needle and insert the needle through the area already anaesthetized. Aspirate as you push forward. The flash back of fluid indicates that you have reached the effusion.

7 Gently aspirate 20 ml of fluid for analysis. Send for:
- Bacteriology: MC&S, ZN stains and TB culture.
- Chemistry: protein, glucose, LDH and amylase.
- Cytology – the more fluid the better (up to 10 ml) as the sample is spun down to concentrate the cells.

8 For therapeutic taps attach a large (white/brown/grey) cannula to a 50 ml syringe and after the flash back of fluid, advance the Venflon slightly and withdraw the needle, leaving the flexible cannula in place. As you do this, ask the patient to breathe out, placing your thumb over the cannula lumen to prevent air being sucked in. Again, ask the patient to breathe out as you attach the three-way tap. Secure the cannula with tape if you are aspirating a large effusion. Attach the 50 ml syringe to one tap, the empty saline bag to the other.

9 Aspirate 50 ml at a time, switching the tap settings to empty the syringe contents into the bowl or saline bag. Do not remove more than 1000 ml at one sitting; more than this can lead to reflex pulmonary oedema.

10 Withdraw the cannula asking the patient to breath out as you do so. Apply an occlusive dressing.

11 CXR is usually only necessary if you have removed a large volume of fluid (>500 ml) or you are concerned about a pneumothorax.

12 Document the procedure, including the macroscopic appearance of the fluid (straw-coloured, blood-stained, containing pus), the volume aspirated, and if you have done (and checked) a CXR.

If you fail

A dry tap indicates a possible loculated effusion or empyema. Try redirecting the needle. If no luck, ask for help from a colleague or radiologist.

Hints

• Ask the patient to cough as you reach the end; this aids in expelling fluid. They usually cough reflexly as the visceral pleura touches the end of the cannula.
• Have a vial of atropine to hand for vaso-vagals (1 ampoule (0.6 mg) IV stat).
• A 'premed' of pethidine (50 mg) IM and prochlorperazine (12.5 mg) IM is very useful for anxious patients.
• Do not take diagnostic samples from the giving set bag (if you use one) as it probably contains a filter that will exclude cellular material.

Pulsus paradoxus

During inspiration, intra-thoracic pressure falls, which reduces the systolic ejection volume and therefore the systolic pressure. Normally, the difference in the systolic pressure during inspiration and expiration is less than 10 mmHg. This pressure difference is exaggerated by a large drop in intra-thoracic pressure that occurs during inhalation in serious conditions, including severe asthma and cardiac tamponade. Pulsus paradoxus is defined by a difference in systolic BP between inspiration and expiration of more than 10 mmHg.

Have ready

A stethoscope and a sphygmomanometer.

The procedure

1 Inflate the cuff above systolic pressure, then slowly deflate until the first, intermittent sounds are heard (during expiration). Note the pressure.
2 Continue to deflate the cuff slowly until the sounds are continuous (i.e. heard during inspiration and expiration). The drop in mmHg between when the first sound is heard (intermittent) and when it becomes continuous represents the degree of paradox.

Respiratory function tests

Spirometry

Have ready

A spirometer, vitalograph paper and a disposable mouthpiece.

The procedure

1 Explain the procedure to the patient and that you need their co-operation.
2 Plug the machine in. Place the vitalograph paper in position on the spirometer. Make sure the spirometer's needle is set to zero. Place the disposable mouthpiece in the end of the spirometer's hosepipe.
3 Ask the patient to take a couple of deep breaths. When ready, ask them to breathe in as deeply as possible and then to breathe all the way out as quickly as possible into the mouthpiece. They

Table 13.4 Expected values for FEV$_1$ (litres).

(a) Males

Age (years)	Height (m)				
	1.50	1.60	1.70	1.80	1.90
15–20	2.80	3.30	3.55	3.90	4.30
20–25	3.25	3.60	3.95	4.35	4.70
25–35	3.10	3.45	3.80	4.20	4.55
35–45	2.80	3.15	3.50	3.90	4.25
45–55	2.50	2.85	3.20	3.60	3.90
55–65	2.15	2.50	2.90	3.25	3.60
65–75	1.85	2.20	2.60	2.95	3.30
75–80	1.55	1.90	2.25	2.65	3.00
85+	1.40	1.75	2.10	2.50	2.85

(b) Females

Age (years)	Height (m)				
	1.40	1.50	1.60	1.70	1.80
15–25	2.45	2.80	3.15	3.45	3.75
25–35	2.35	2.65	2.95	3.30	3.65
35–45	2.05	2.35	2.65	3.05	3.35
45–55	1.75	2.05	2.35	2.75	3.05
55–65	1.45	1.75	2.10	2.45	2.75
65–75	1.15	1.45	1.85	2.15	2.45
75–80	0.85	1.20	1.55	1.85	2.15
85+	0.75	1.05	1.35	1.70	2.05

Table 13.5 Expected normal values for FVC (litres).

(a) Males

Age (years)	Height (m)				
	1.50	1.60	1.70	1.80	1.90
15–20	3.45	4.00	4.50	5.05	5.55
20–25	3.65	4.15	4.70	5.20	5.75
25–35	3.55	4.05	4.60	5.10	5.60
35–45	3.30	3.85	4.35	4.90	5.40
45–55	3.10	3.60	4.15	4.65	5.20
55–65	2.85	3.40	3.95	4.45	4.95
65–75	2.65	3.15	3.70	4.20	4.75
75–80	2.45	2.95	3.45	4.00	4.50
85+	2.35	2.85	3.35	3.90	4.40

(b) Females

Age (years)	Height (m)				
	1.50	1.60	1.70	1.80	1.90
15–25	2.90	3.40	3.85	4.35	4.75
25–35	2.75	3.25	3.70	4.15	4.65
35–45	2.45	2.95	3.45	3.90	4.35
45–55	2.20	2.65	3.15	3.60	4.05
55–65	1.90	2.35	2.85	3.30	3.75
65–75	1.60	2.10	2.55	3.00	3.45
75–80	1.30	1.80	2.25	2.70	3.20
85+	1.20	1.65	2.10	2.60	3.05

Table 13.6 Predicted values for PEFR (litre/minute).

(a) Males

Age (years)	Height (m)				
	1.50	1.60	1.70	1.80	1.90
15–20	440	475	510	545	580
20–25	535	570	610	645	680
25–35	525	560	595	630	665
35–45	500	535	570	605	635
45–55	480	510	545	575	610
55–65	455	490	520	550	580
65–75	435	465	495	525	550
75–80	410	440	465	495	525
85+	410	430	455	480	510

(b) Females

Age (years)	Height (m)				
	1.50	1.60	1.70	1.80	1.90
15–25	360	395	435	470	510
25–35	350	385	420	460	495
35–45	325	365	400	440	475
45–55	305	345	380	420	455
55–65	285	320	360	395	435
65–75	265	300	340	375	415
75–80	245	280	315	355	390
85+	235	270	305	345	380

should breathe out until the needle reaches the end of the graph paper.

4 Depending on how automated the machine is, you may need to push the record button while the patient is exhaling.

5 Repeat a few times, particularly if the first attempt(s) are feeble.

6 Record the best FEV_1 and FVC in the notes, with expected values for the patient (see Tables 13.4 & 13.5):

The patient has a restrictive picture if FVC is reduced and $FEV_1/FVC > 75\%$.

The patient has an obstructive picture if $FEV_1/FVC < 75\%$.

Peak expiratory flow rate

Measures the maximum expiratory flow rate in the first 2 ms of expiration, and is useful for assessing the respiratory status of patients with asthma, COAD and other respiratory conditions, especially before surgery.

Have ready

A peak flow meter and disposable mouthpiece.

The procedure

1 Put the disposable mouthpiece into the peak flow meter.

2 Ask the patient to breathe in as deeply as possible.

3 With their lips tightly sealed around the mouthpiece, ask them to blow out forcefully and quickly. Note the value attained.

4 Have them repeat it at least three times.

5 Record the best value in the notes, with the expected value (Table 13.6).

Sutures

You may be expected to do simple suturing. The method is best learnt in A&E or in theatre. Ask someone to teach you how to tie a basic, non-slip knot as soon as you can. Table 13.7 discusses times for suture removal.

Materials

1 Non-absorbable
  • Nylon (ethilon).
  • Ethibond.

Table 13.7 When to remove sutures.

Area sutured	Removal time (days)
Face and neck	3–5
Scalp	5–7
Abdomen and chest	5–10
If impaired wound healing (steroids, cachexia, severe infection etc.)	14 or more

- Prolene**.
- Silk**.

2 Absorbable
- Plain cat gut (5–10 days).
- Chromic gut (10–20 days).
- Vicryl (60–90 days)**.
- Dexon (60–90 days)**

3 Sizes
- Very coarse – 2, 1, 0, 1/0, 2/0, etc.
Very fine – 6/0, 5/0, etc.
- 3/0 and 4/0 are suitable for skin on arms and legs.
- 5/0 and 6/0 for face and back of the hand.
- 2/0 is most often used for securing lines and 1/0 for chest drains.

4 Needles
Either use a cutting needle (with a bev-
elled edge) for suturing skin or a non-cutting needle (with a rounded end) for adipose and other soft tissues.

Hints

- Nylon is less comfortable for patients. Use softer, non-absorbable material (silk or prolene) for securing lines and chest drains.
- Some synthetic sutures are made as mono or polyfilament. Monofilament sutures are more slippery, but are better if there is a high risk of infection. Polyfilament sutures facilitate tracking of fluid down the suture, leading to infection.

** Most commonly used for House Officer purposes.

Chapter 14: Radiology

Radiologists can help you a great deal with patient management if you give them enough information.

Most of the following guidelines come from the Royal College of Radiologists.[1] Your hospital may also have its own.

Requesting investigations

1 Always book procedures as early as possible. Most radiological departments are over-booked. This is particularly true for contrast studies, CTs and MRIs.

2 Include lots of information on the X-ray form, such as:
- Patient ID.
- Whether pregnant or not. Any reactions to contrast media.
- A specific question to be answered.
- Clinical features (not just suspected diagnosis).
- Any factors which may complicate the procedure (e.g. diabetes, epilepsy).
- 'Please' and 'Thank you' go a long way.

3 Ask the radiographers about how to prepare patients for investigations, such as barium enemas. Often the radio-

grapher will liaise directly with the ward nurse, in which case you don't have to do anything except prescribe preparations, such as enemas (see below). However, it's good to find out about the different preparations so that you can tell patients in advance what they are letting themselves in for. Better still, try them yourself – you will never order a barium meal lightly again!

Minimizing radiation

- 27% of the radiation we are exposed to comes from radiological sources.
- In terms of radiation, different procedures are ranked as indicated in Table 14.1.

Common concerns about X-rays

Patients are usually concerned about being X-rayed. It is much kinder to address their likely concerns outright. Therefore, wherever possible, tell the patient:

1 What is about to happen to them.
2 Why they are having this done.
3 How long it might take.
4 Whether or not they will be sedated or have a general anaesthetic.
5 The amount and type of pain and discomfort to expect.
6 What to do if they have pain or other symptoms after the procedure.

[1] RCR Working Party (1993). *Making the Best use of a Department of Clinical Radiology: Guidelines for Doctors.* 2nd edn. The Royal College of Radiologists, London.

Table 14.1 Radiation doses of radiological investigations.

Investigation	Radiation dose (mSv)	Number of CXRs
Abdomen	1.5	75
Barium–oesophagus study	2	100
Barium–small bowel study	6	300
Barium–stomach study	5	250
Biliary tract	1.3	65
Cervical spine	0.1	5
Chest film	0.02	1
CT chest/abdomen	8	400
CT head	2	100
Dorsal spine	1.0	50
Extremities (e.g. knee)	0.01	0.5
Hip (one)	0.3	15
IVU	4.6	230
Large bowel study	9	450
Lumbar spine	2.4	120
Nuclear study bone	3.8	190
Nuclear study kidney	0.7	35
Nuclear study liver	0.7	35
Nuclear study lung	1.2	60
Nuclear study myocardium	18	900
Nuclear study thyroid	1	50
Pelvic plain film	1	50

RCR working party (1993). *Making the Best Use of a Department of Clinical Radiology: Guidelines for Doctors*. 2nd edn. The Royal College of Radiologists, London.

7 When they can eat/drink/drive/talk/have sex.

8 Whether they will have any scars or permanent after effects.

9 Who is doing the procedure.

Pregnancy

• Referring clinicians (i.e. you) are responsible for informing the radiologist if a patient is pregnant. Notify the radiologist clearly on the X-ray form. It is negligent not to do this. Where possible tell the radiologist yourself.

• If you need to X-ray a pregnant patient, ask the radiologist for advice; they may suggest an alternative. Irradiation between the knees and diaphragm should be avoided.

Plain films

Chest X-rays before surgery

'Routine' CXRs are warranted pre-operatively if the patient has:

• Chronic heart or lung disease and no CXR within 12 months.

• Acute respiratory symptoms.

• Known/suspected malignant disease.

• Possible TB.

Age, smoking and mild hypertension are *not* reasons for routine chest X-rays.

Checking the CXR: the bare bones

1 Patients name and the date of the film.

2 Trace the diaphragm and the lateral outline of the rib cage (? pleural effusions, air under the diaphram, raised hemi-diaphragm, pneumothorax).

3 Check the size and shape of the heart (? enlarged heart, atrial shadows, calcified valve rings).

4 Check the position of trachea and heart (? displaced or is the film rotated).

5 Look at the mediastinum (? air, widened, lymphadenpathy).

6 Examine the hilar shadows (? enlarged pulmonary arteries and veins).

7 Examine the lungs (? opacities – consolidation, fluid or nodules). For interstitial edema remember to look for straight lines (normal interstitial shadows are 'never' straight).

8 Check the bony structures (ribs, clavicles, spine) and the soft tissues (fractures, densities or lucencies, air in the tissues).

Skull X-rays

You rarely need to X-ray someone's skull following a head injury. A CT is the investigation of choice. The Royal College's guidelines are shown in Table 14.2.

• To differentiate CSF from normal nasal or aural discharge in a patient with head injury, test it with a urine dipstick. CSF contains glucose.

Abdominal films

Radiation dose: 75 CXRs.

Preparation:

• None.

Tell the radiologist:

• Presenting symptoms (not just 'acute abdomen').

• Past surgery.

• Pregnancy.

• Ask for an erect film if you need to check fluid levels.

Tell the patient:

• Quick, minimal irradiation.

A decubitus film is an alternative to

Table 14.2 Royal College guidelines regarding skull X-rays.

SKULL X-RAY NOT INDICATED *All of the following:* • Full orientation • Neurologically normal • No scalp laceration or haematoma • Amnesia <10 minutes	MANAGEMENT • Request neurological observation 6-hourly from the nurses (if already an inpatient) *or* have relatives take home a head injury form
SKULL X-RAY OR CT INDICATED *Full orientation plus any one or more of following:* • Serious scalp laceration • Scalp haematoma (90% are associated with fracture) • Clinical signs of closed fracture • Known loss of consciousness • Amnesia >10 minutes • Evidence of foreign body • Evidence of penetrating injury	MANAGEMENT • CT is the invesigation of choice. Unless you are expert at reading skull X-rays show a skull X-ray to a senior before going to bed
SKULL X-RAY OR CT *One or more of the following:* • Disorientated or worse • Difficult to assess; drunk	MANAGEMENT • Admit for observation • Consult with neurosurgeons if fracture evident *or* no improvement in 12 hours

an erect CXR to see perforation if the patient is too ill to sit up

Checking an abdominal plain film

1 Patients name and date of the film; whether taken erect, supine (usual) or lateral decubitus.
2 Gas pattern; intestinal diameter: small bowel > 2.5 cm, or colon > 6 cm indicates obstruction.
3 Look for ascites and soft tissue masses. ? Oedema in the intestinal wall. Faecal distribution.
4 Identify the liver and spleen.
5 Check the borders of the kidneys, bladder and psoas muscles if possible.
6 Calculi (gall stones, renal and pancreatic calculi, aortic calcification).

7 Sub-diaphragmatic gas (or clear outline of organ) indicates perforation or recent surgery. (Note: sub-diaphragmatic gas is best seen on an erect CXR.

Contrast studies

Intravenous urography

Radiation dose: 230 CXRs.
Preparation:
• Picolax (1 sachet) 12–24 hours before the procedure (not essential).
• Preferably NBM 6 hours before.
• Keep well hydrated before and after, to minimize contrast nephrotoxicity; give IV fluids if necessary.

Tell radiologist:
• If patient has renal damage, diabetes or myeloma.
• Contrast allergy or pregnancy.
Tell patient:
• Warn about preparation.

Barium swallow

Radiation dose: 100 CXRs.
Preparation:
• NBM 6 hours before.
Tell the radiologist:
• Oesophageal disease or surgery.
• Contrast allergy or pregnancy.
Tell the patient:
• Quick, painless but tastes horrible!

Barium meal

Radiation dose: 250 CXRs.
Preparation:
• NBM 6 hours before.
Tell the radiologist:
• Upper GI disease or surgery.
• Contrast allergy or pregnancy.
Tell the patient:
• Painless but tastes awful.

Small bowel enema

Radiation dose: 300 CXRs.
Preparation:
• 24 hours low residue diet.
• Laxative (e.g. 1 sachet of Picolax) 24 and 12 hours prior to procedure *unless* contraindicated (e.g. IBD, PR bleeding); get radiologist's advice.
Tell the radiologist:
• Past surgery.
• Contrast allergy or pregnancy.
Tell the patient:
• Warn them about diet and laxative.
• Takes at least half an hour; may take 2 hours.

• Uncomfortable; requires upper GI intubation.

Barium enema

Radiation dose: 450 CXRs.
Contraindication:
• Severe colonic inflammation (e.g. IBD, severe diverticulitis) and toxic megacolon.
Preparation:
• Do not perform immediately prior to CT abdomen/chest (barium hides detail on CT for at least 72 hours). Do the CT first or consider using gastrograffin.
• Book for >72 hours after rectal biopsy and rigid sigmoidoscopy to avoid perforation.
• Strong laxative 24 and 12 hours before procedure *unless* acute IBD; ask radiologist for advice.
Tell the radiologist:
• Previous surgery.
• Contrast allergy or pregnancy.
• Result of sigmoidoscopy/rectal biopsy/rectal exam.
Tell the patient:
• Warn them of diet and laxative.
• Procedure takes 20–30 minutes.
• Pictures will be taken every 10–15 minutes while the patient is turned around on a platform. The procedure is *very* undignified, uncomfortable and often upsetting.

Ultrasound

No radiation or contraindications.
Preparation:
• Abdominal US: NBM 6 hours before.
• Pelvic US: Requires full bladder.
• The patient should start drinking a few hours before the procedure.

Tell the patient:
• No radiation dose or known hazards; painless, relatively quick.

Computerized tomography

Preparation:
• Nil unless contrast is needed – ask the radiologist.
Tell the radiologist:
• Any metalwork *in situ* (difficult to interpret).
Tell the patient:
• Will be confined in a noisy tube.
• Painless; will be told what to do by the doctor and nurse.

General

• CTs give large radiation doses (400 CXRs equivalents for abdominal and chest CTs and 100 for skull CTs). Does the patient really need one?
• Usually hospital CTs are over-booked, so book your patient in as early as possible.
• Do CTs *before* requesting barium studies. Barium hides detail on CT and takes at least 3 days to clear. Gastrograffin can be used instead of barium if this is a problem.
• Patients may require sedation before CT; 10 mg of temazepam 30 minutes before the procedure is usually adequate.

CT head – indications

Stroke: diagnosis in doubt; atypical clinical course; to differentiate haem-orrhage from infarct if planning anticoagulation. Must be done within 2 weeks for accurate differentiation.

Sub-arachnoid haemorrhage: to exclude a raised ICP before doing an LP; for diagnosis; to diagnose the cause of deterioration (re-bleed, hydrocephalus, vascular spasm).

Head injury: skull fracture and serious scalp injury; impaired consciousness; focal neurology; epilepsy; persistent confusion; deteriorating conscious level; depressed skull fracture; open skull fracture of vault or base.

Arteriography

Preparation:
• Nil to eat for 6 hours before; nothing to drink 3 hours before.
• G&S; FBC (specifically platelets); INR; find both femoral pulses.
• Keep well hydrated before and after to minimize contrast nephrotoxicity; give IV fluids if necessary.
• If patient has renal damage, diabetes or myeloma, discuss with radiologist.
Tell the radiologist:
• Contrast allergy or pregnancy.
Tell the patient:
• The radiologist will numb the skin in the groin and then inject some dye into the artery. They may get a bruise.

Magnetic resonance imaging

• MRI does not emit ionizing radiation but scans are formidably expensive (approximately £400 per scan). Does your patient really need one?
• Book your patient in as early as possible and discuss the procedure with radiologist.

• Pacemakers and *any kind of metal insertion* are an absolute contraindication to MRI.

• T1 weighted images give good anatomical detail. Fat is white, flowing blood is black. T2 images are good at showing abnormal tissue but have poor anatomical detail. Fat and fluid are bright.

Preparation:

• Sedation may be necessary (usually given by the radiologist).

Tell the radiologist:

• If the patient is pregnant.

• METAL INSERTIONS ARE A CONTRAINDICATION FOR MRI.

Tell the patient:

• No irradiation is used. The procedure is painless.

• The patient will be in a noisy, confined space for approximately 25 minutes, although it may seem longer.

Radioisotope scanning

Use to detect:

1 Bony metastases and sites of inflammation – technetium (Tm) scanning.

• Radioisotope scanning delivers variable radiation doses. Ensure that the patient is not pregnant.

• Most scanning does not require preparation, but as usual, book early.

2 Pulmonary embolism – ventilation perfusion (VQ) scans.

• There is no preparation for a VQ scan. These are usually done once a week, so make sure you book one well in advance.

Chapter 15: Surgery

Looking after surgical patients is not intrinsically difficult, but it does involve a lot of running around. You will accompany surgeons on many rapid ward rounds weekly. Have a piece of paper ready for the tasks that will be fired at you from all directions. Overall, the essential thing is timing—if nothing else, make sure you have patients and results ready for theatre.

Routine clerking

House Officers must make sure that patients are fit for surgery. While clerking routine surgical patients can be mundane, it is useful to bear in mind that you may be the only one able to detect medical problems before the patient goes to theatre.

• *Before you see the patient*, quickly flick through the notes (summaries are particularly useful) to give yourself an idea of what has happened previously. This will reassure the patient and helps you to fill in their past medical history.

• Clerking patients before nurses have finished their admission routine is sure to create havoc. Ask the nurse to let you know when s/he has finished.

• Take everything you need to finish clerking to the bedside:
  Sticky labels.
  History sheets (see below).
  Consent form.
  Drug chart.
  Fluid chart.
  Blood bottles and forms: (FBC, C&E, G&S or cross-match, +/− INR +/− glucose).
  IV cannulae.

• Find out how to order sticky labels and order them whenever they look like they are running short on a patient. Writing patient details on endless forms and bottles is no fun.

History sheet
1 Operation (e.g. 'For TURP'), last meal, LMP
2 Past surgical history
3 Past medical history (HASH CREDIT*)
4 Medications and CASES**
5 *Allergies* (very important—especially past drug reactions to anaesthesia)
6 Home care (lives with, home help, family diseases, mobility)
7 Functional enquiry: CVS, RS, GIT, GU, CNS, MSK
8 Examination
9 Impression
10 Differential diagnoses
11 Plan

---

*HASH CREDIT: **H**ypertension, **A**sthma /COAD, **S**ickle cell, **H**IV/Hepatitis, **C**VA, **R**F, **E**pilepsy, **D**iabetes, **I**schaemic Heart Disease, **T**B. Alternatively, SHIRC DEATH, HEH DRASTIC.
CASES: **Contraception, **A**nticoagulants, **S**teroids, **E**toh/alcohol, **S**moking.

• Make your own protocol clerking sheet, custom-designed for your specialty (see Fig. 15.1, p. 190). If useful, include the boxed pre-op anaesthetist checklist (p. 184). To photocopy the protocol onto real history sheets, write or type it out on a blank sheet of paper lined up with a history sheet, and then feed real history sheets into the photocopying machine.

• If you have literally 3 minutes to clerk a patient, at least make sure that a) the patient has the problem that they are supposed to have; b) they are fit for surgery. You may be the only person that checks them for cardiovascular and respiratory problems.

• G&S or cross-match patients ahead of time. It is wise to routinely G&S virtually all patients on admission if you haven't already cross-matched them. If necessary you can then phone the blood bank to cross-match them quickly (in 30 minutes). Unless you ask the lab to hold onto it for longer, G&S blood is usually thrown out after 3 days and may need to be repeated (see Table 15.1).

Table 15.1 Preparations for different operations.

Operation	G&S/cross-match	Special needs
Abdominoperineal repair/AP resection	4	Prepare for stoma
Amputation (minor) Amputation (major)	G&S 2+	Pain +/– grief Fentanyl and clonidine infusion works well; buscopan helps muscular contracture pain
Aneurysm repair (elective)	6	Post-op ITU
Aneurysm repair (emergency)	10	Post-op ITU
Aortobifemoral repair	6	
Appendicectomy	G&S	Metronidazole PR post-op saves a drip
Arthroscopy	Nil	
Carotid endarterectomy	2	
Cholecystectomy	G&S	
Colectomy	2	Prepare for stoma
Dynamic hip screw	2	Be alert to post-op infection
ERCP	G&S	Pre-op abdominal US Post-op amylase

continued on p. 180

Table 15.1 (*continued*)

Operation	G&S/cross-match	Special needs
Femoropopliteal repair	2	
Gastrectomy	2	Bad pain post-op; try continuous morphine infusion
Hemi-arthoplasty	2	
Hernia	Nil	
Ileal reservoir	2	
Laparotomy	2	Consent for colostomy/ileostomy
Liver biopsy	G&S	Pre-op INR (see p. 118)
Liver/pancreatic surgery	6	Post-op amylase
Mastectomy	G&S	Prepare for grief over loss of breasts and body image and get a prosthesis nurse to talk to the patient Drains in for several days (remove when they have stopped discharging)
Oesophagectomy	4	
Prostatectomy (TURP)	2–4	Watch for post-op haemorrhage (look for bad haematuria). May need to cross-match more blood post-op
Pyloric stenosis	G&S	
Splenectomy	2	Pre-op pneumococcal +/− HiB, +/− meningococcal vaccines
Thyroidectomy	2–4	Pre-op vocal cord assessment from ENT clinic post-op Ca check
Total hip replacement	4	Watch for DVT/PE and infection; usually routine anticoagulation required
TURT	G&S	Pre-op MSU
Varicose veins	G&S	

• Check local transfusion requirements for specific operations.

• ITU can be a frightening place. Try to organize for patients undergoing major operations to meet ITU staff or visit the ITU before theatre in preparation for their post-op stay. Nurses will often organize this for you.

• Do a sickle cell test on black patients if their haematological status is unknown.

• Patients must be NBM for solids for at least 6 hours before going to theatre, and 3 hours for sips of liquid. This is a fairly strict rule. In a real emergency anaesthetists do 'crash induction'. Discuss this if necessary with the anaesthetist.

Peri-operative prescribing

• Prescribe as much as possible during the clerking, as it saves time later: regular drugs; pre-medication; prophylactic antibiotics; prophylactic heparin; analgesia; routine post-op antibiotics (consider PR administration to save IVs); extra steroids if the patient takes them already (to overcome post-op stress).

• Check the firm's use of prophylactic antibiotics and anticoagulants.

• 20 mg temazepam orally with a small sip of water can be used as a pre-med if necessary. This can usually be given within an hour of theatre, although it should be given 3 hours before. Check with the anaesthetist if in doubt.

• A fentanyl infusion can be effective pain relief (less side effects than morphine but more expensive; problems appear within first 10–15 minutes).

• Patients should have stopped taking non-steroidals and anticoagulants *at least* a week (preferably a month) before

surgery. If they have not, ask your senior or anaesthetist for your firm's policy on how to proceed. The effects of anticoagulants fall within days of stopping them and usually you can cover patients with FFP. Patients with artificial heart valves or other conditions requiring continuous anticoagulation should be switched over to heparin – consult your seniors.

• The *BNF* recommends that people stop taking the oral contraceptive pill at least 4 weeks before major surgery. If the patient has not done this, consider IV or SC heparin before surgery, but check with the anaesthetist or surgeon first. The pill does not need to be stopped for minor surgery such as laparoscopic sterilization. Progestagen-only pills do not need to be stopped.

Consent

Criteria for valid consent[1]
1 No coercion
2 Patient informed
3 Patient competent

However rushed you are, patients must understand major and common hazards and discomforts of the procedure they are about to undergo. *Note*: Legally you may only obtain consent for a procedure you have personally performed. However, the situation 'on the ground' is very different and seniors often expect you to 'take consent'. Refuse except to give the patient information in advance

[1] Hope R.A. *et al.* (1994). *Oxford Practice Skills Project: sample teaching materials.* Oxford Medical School, Oxford.

of the operator getting informed consent (to make their job easier).

• If you will perform the procedure yourself (like a bone marrow biopsy), never get consent if you do not know all the risks or logistics of the procedure. If in doubt ask you senior.

• While taking consent, you can spend a few minutes improving the patient's understanding of their overall course of management (not just the procedure). This is a good opportunity to develop a relationship with the patient.

• A signature alone does not stand in a court of law as adequate proof of consent. The patient must understand the procedure.

• Make sure you get parental consent for minors while the parents are on the ward, or you will have to call them in from home. ('Minors' are people under 16 years of age.) Occasionally it may be lawful to treat a child under sixteen without parental consent, but you must be sure that he or she fully understands the treatment, that his/her health would be likely to suffer without treatment, that you have attempted to persuade the child to involve their parents, and that you are sure it is in the childs best interest to proceed without informing the parents. You must get senior advice in these situations. Rarely, parents refuse consent to treatment that their child needs. Unless it is an acute situation, an application will be necessary through the hospital's solicitors or Social Services.

• Diagrams can save many words. If you are in a specialty where you need consent for a particular procedure many times, a well-constructed diagram can save you a lot of time in the long run.

Photocopy it and leave it with the patient.

• Remember that while *you* may understand anatomical diagrams, the patient may not. Sometimes a conceptual diagram is more useful, if not as accurate. See Appendix B for diagrams which you can use to explain standard procedures to your patients.

• Check with nurses to see if your department has information sheets already made up which you can give to patients.

• Always consent patients undergoing laparoscopic surgery for open surgery. (5–10% of patients undergoing laparoscopic cholecystectomy end up having open surgery.)

• Always consider consenting patients undergoing bowel resection or laparoscopy for colostomy/ileostomy in case they need one. (Write '+/− colostomy/ileostomy' on the consent form.) Warn them that this may happen and arrange with the nurses for a stoma nurse to see them.

In all cases of surgery it is important to inform patients of :

• Fatigue. It is important to tell patients to expect to feel quite low and very tired for several weeks post-op (1–3 months for major surgery).

• Anaesthetic risk. Although the anaesthetist will consent for the anaesthetic, it is a good idea to ask whether or not the patient has had any previous adverse reactions.

• Bleeding. Reassure patients that major bleeding is very uncommon (they often fear it the most). However, it is a risk they should be aware of.

• Infection.

• Advise about the likelihood of waking up with drains from the wound, an O_2 mask and NGT. Drains and NGT may stay in place for several days. Advise also that post-op nausea from the anaesthetic is possible and that post-op pain will be treated.

Expected side effects after surgery

Amputation. Sloughing; cramps; phantom pain; psychological distress; need for revision.

Aortic aneurysm repair. Bleeding; thrombo-embolism; ureteric damage; paraplegia (from anterior spinal artery damage); gut ischaemia; ARDS; renal failure; aorto-enteric fistula. Also fatigue and feeling low. These patients usually go to ITU post-op.

Biliary surgery. Jaundice; strictures; pancreatitis; hepato-renal syndrome; bleeding. Drainage tubes in place.

Abdominal/colonic surgery. Constipation (ileus); fistulae; anastomotic leaks; obstruction; trauma to ureters. The patient will need counselling about a stoma; contact your stoma nurse to arrange this if the nurses have not already done so. Always consent patients undergoing colonic surgery for ileostomy/colostomy and warn them that they may have one when they wake up.

Genito-urinary surgery. Ureteral and renal damage. Infection.

Mastectomy. Arm oedema; anxiety/depression.

Splenectomy. Infection (pneumococcal septicaemia); thrombocytosis. The patient should have been given pn-

eumococcal, HiB +/− meningococcal vaccines at least 1 week prior to surgery; if not, they need it. Consult immediately with seniors. Splenectomized patients need prophylactic antibiotics (penicillin V 250–500 mg bd) probably for the rest of their lives (people have died of pneumococcal sepsis 20 years post-op). They will also need advice about coping with the side effects of antibiotics (diarrhoea, candidiasis, particularly vaginal thrush). They also need a card and preferably a medical bracelet to alert others that they have no spleen.

Thyroid surgery. Bleeding; hoarseness (laryngeal nerve palsy).

Tracheostomy. Stenosis; mediastinitis; surgical emphysema.

Prostatectomy. Urinary retention post-op; urethral stricture and incontinence; bleeding; retrograde ejaculation (usually asymptomatic but important to mention!).

Haemorrhoidectomy. Bleeding and anal stricture.

Anaesthetics

Make friends with your firm's anaesthetist. Anaesthetists usually come to see patients (and you) the evening before theatre. Having everything ready for them saves a lot of headaches.
• Get an anaesthetic rota from the anaesthetic department. This saves telephone calls when you need to find the anaesthetist to warn them of late changes or patient complications.
• Tell your anaesthetist about a) late

changes to a patient or procedure, b) high risk patients.

• Check whether you or the anaesthetist need to prescribe the premedication.

• Arrange for ECGs to be done on admission for anyone older than 50.

• Arrange for CXRs to be done on patients well in time for theatre as local protocols require (routine pre-op CXRs are not recommended by the Royal College of Radiologists, see p. 173).

• Arrange for neck X-rays to be done on patients with rheumatoid arthritis.

• Write a checklist in the notes for patients going to theatre. The following is routine, but add or subtract lines depending on your specialty.

Pre-op checklist
Premed – prescribed/given . . . .
NBM for x hours . . . .
FBC: . . . .
C&E: . . . .
ECG – done/NA . . . .
CXR + report . . . .
(No) sickle cell disease, liver disease, COAD, CVS disease . . . .
(No) allergies . . . .
Special needs: . . . .

• Have the anaesthetist help you to insert cannulae if you have trouble. It is much less stressful putting them into unconscious patients.

• Ask the anaesthetist to teach you how to intubate patients.

Drawing up theatre lists

Some hospitals require House Officers to do this.

• Include: Name of the surgeon to do each case.

Name of the theatre.

Date and time the list is supposed to start.

Name, sex, age, hospital number and ward of each patient.

Procedure.

Special information (e.g. high risk status).

• Put children and diabetics first.

• Put 'dirty' (bowel) surgery and high risk patients last.

• Let theatre staff know that a patient is high risk so they can get prepared.

Marking patients for surgery

• Use an indelible pen and mark boldly.

• Discuss varicose vein marking with the surgeon.

Post-operative care

Post-op patients are usually much less work than pre-op patients. However, be alert to post-op emergencies as well as slow onset complications. PEs, stress-induced heart failure, MI, haemorrhage, anaesthetic and steroid reactions, as well as terrible pain all require urgent action. It is *vital* to remember emergency routines for these problems, even if you do not use them much during your surgical rotation. Nursing staff on surgical convalescent wards may not know much about medical emergencies and it may be up to you to start rapid treatment.

1 It is a good idea to conduct your own daily ward round, particularly if you are on call for the evening. Dunn and

Rawlinson provide a useful ward round checklist that enables you to take command of your ward[2]:

- Ask the patient about pain, breathing, eating, bowels and bladder output.
- Examine the chest, abdomen, wound, legs, mental state.
- Check drains, lines and catheters for drainage and local infection. Are they still necessary?
- Look at the charts for pyrexia, tachycardia and changes in BP and fluid balance.
- Make sure the patient is written up for adequate analgesia, night sedation, antibiotics and fluids. Are they all still necessary?
- Order investigations:
  - FBC, C&E post-op.
  - C&E daily for as long as the patient is on a drip.
  - Other tests to check for specific complications of different operations.

2 Remember to look for the '4W' complications: Wound, Walking, Wind, Water (i.e. wound infection, DVT, chest infection/PE and poor urine output). Ileus is also a common problem.

Complicated patients

Jaundice

Problems: excessive bleeding and dehydration, resulting in hepato-renal syndrome if pre-existing liver disease.
Do:

[2] Dunn D.C. & Rawlinson N. (1991). *Surgical Diagnosis and Management: A Guide to General Surgical Care.* Blackwell Science, Oxford.

- Pre- and post-op liver function tests, INR and KCCT.
- Avoid morphine in pre-medication.
- Ensure adequate IV fluids. Hydrate pre-op if necessary (care if heart failure, ascites or low albumin). Use 5% dextrose, not saline.
Consider:
- Pre-op vitamin K.
- Pre-op renal dose dopamine.
- Post-op 2-hourly urine output check.
- Post-op IV fluids to match fluid losses (urine, NGT, stool).
- Measure C&E daily.
- Avoid saline if the person is in liver failure and has ascites.

Diabetes

Problems: hypoglycaemia; ketoacidosis precipitated by stress and dehydration; post-op infection. Also, this group has a high percentage of silent MIs. For surgical protocol see Table 15.2.

For all diabetics

- Consider ECG.
- Check local protocols.

For well-controlled NIDDM

- Do pre-op fasting glucose (preferably the day before surgery).
- If pre-op fasting glucose is greater than 11 U, halve the oral hypoglycaemic dose the day before surgery and omit the oral hypoglycaemic on the day of surgery.
- If pre-op fasting glucose is greater than 11 U, follow the IDDM regime in Table 15.2.
- For minor procedures and even larger procedures if the patient is eating on the same day, simply omit the morning

Table 15.2 Surgical protocols for people with diabetes.

	Minor surgery (eating same day)	Major surgery, especially GI (not eating for several days)
Well-controlled NIDDM	• Omit morning hypoglycaemic drugs	• Omit hypoglycaemic drugs • Monitor blood glucose qds • GKI/sliding scale if insulin needed
Poorly controlled NIDDM and IDDM	• Omit morning insulin • Monitor blood glucose • Return to usual regime as soon as eating • NIDDM may need insulin on a PRN basis	• Keep on GKI/IV sliding scale/qds insulin until eating

Table 15.3 The GKI (Glucose, Potassium, Insulin) regime—as used in Newcastle

500 ml of 10% dextrose with 10 mmol KCl and variable insulin, usually 12–16 units Actrapid. Infuse at 80 ml/hour

If blood glucose 7–10 continue
If blood glucose > 10 and rising, put up a new bag containing 4 more units of insulin than previously
If blood glucose < 7, use a new bag with 4 units *less* insulin
Blood glucose < 3 give 200 ml 10% dextrose and re-check the blood glucose

The rationale of this regime is that it provides both insulin and dextrose. It thus suppresses ketone production and avoids problems that might occur with separate insulin and glucose infusions, such as the glucose drip finishing or blocking while the insulin drip carries on, potentially causing hypoglycaemia

hypoglycaemic. Institute IV insulin/ GKI (Table 15.3) if uncontrolled (BM > 10).
• If the patient is undergoing major surgery, follow the GKI and omit the oral hypoglycaemic agent on the day of surgery.

For IDDM and poorly controlled NIDDM

• Put the patient first on the list and tell the surgeon (or theatre sister) that the patient is diabetic.

• Pre-op fasting glucose, urea, C&E, FBC (at least).
• Ensure good IV access pre-op (at least a green cannula).
• If the operation is in the morning, omit all insulin or hypoglycaemic drugs.
• Use the GKI regime (see Table 15.3).

Insulin infusion

• Draw up 50 units of short-acting insulin (e.g. Actrapid) in a 50 ml syringe and then fill the syringe with 50 ml of normal saline. This means that there is 1

Table 15.4 Insulin sliding scale.

Fingerprick glucose (mmol)	IV soluble insulin (units/hour)
<2	None. Give 50 ml of 50% glucose. Call doctor
4.0–6.4	0.5
6.5–8.9	1
9.0–10.9	2
11.0–16.9	3
17.0–28.0	4
>28	8 Call doctor

unit of insulin/ml, allowing easy adjustment according to the sliding scale shown in Table 15.4.

• Label the syringe (see p. 97).

• Set up an infusion pump (p. 97) or put the syringe in the fridge and let the nurses know where it is.

• To convert this scale to a SC scale, give four times the IV dose. This is because SC insulin is given every 4 hours instead of every hour.

• Work out how much insulin the patient normally receives, in whatever form. For example, if s/he gets a total of 100 units/24 hours as a mixture of long and short acting insulin, then adjust the sliding scale so that roughly 100 units of short acting insulin is given over 24 hours. However, you will need to reduce the normal dose while the patient is not eating.

• Make sure you check C&E at least once daily while the patient is on a sliding scale of insulin and a K infusion. Adjust K accordingly. Remember that K comes out of cells as blood glucose rises and can suddenly drop if the patient's glucose comes under control.

• If the fingerprick glucose is persistently >11, increase each insulin dose on the sliding scale by 0.5–1.0 units. On the other hand, if the fingerprick glucose is constantly < 4.0 mM reduce each insulin dose on the sliding scale by 0.5–1.0 units.

Steroid-dependent patients

(see The steroid patient p. 110)

Problem: risk of life theatening hypotension (Addisionian crisis). Steroid dependent patients need extra steroid cover for surgical stress.

• Ensure good IV access.

• Major surgery: give 100 mg hydrocortisone IM/IV with pre-med, then 6-hourly for 3 days.

• Minor surgery: as above, but only give post-op hydrocortisone for 24 hours.

Thyroid surgery

Problems: vocal chord damage, post-op thyroid storm, bleeding.

• Have vocal chords checked by ENT pre-op.

• Cross-match at least 2–4 units pre-op *and* G&S post-op.

• Ensure good IV access.

• Measure Ca post-op.

• Patients who have undergone thyroid surgery should have clip removers at the bedside. If they bleed suddenly the surgical clips should be removed to prevent suffocation and to allow the bleeding to be controlled directly with pressure.

Day surgery

More and more operations are being done as day surgery; the Royal College of Surgeons' target is 50%.

• Don't spend too much time clerking day surgery patients (usually 5–10 minutes). They have usually been checked over at least twice already. However, you do need to ensure they have no obvious CVS or respiratory problems (like a recent cold), and if necessary, to send them home.

• Develop a protocol clerking sheet for your day patients (see p. 189).

• Prescribe adequate take-home analgesia. Poor pain relief is the most common problem for patients—and for GPs who have to prescribe it.[3] A few paracetamol are not adequate postoperatively. Co-proxamol (2 tabs) 4–6-hourly is standard, but check with your surgeons and the nursing staff.

• Tell patients what to expect, especially within the first 24 hours. For instance, fatigue and wound-related discomfort are normal. Tell patients that you are giving them pain killers to take home with them and that they should use them!

• Tell patients:

They can't drive for 48 hours and they certainly can't drive home.

They can eat and drink.

They should have a contact number for the hospital and their GP should any problems arise (it is helpful to give the hospital day surgery contact number to patients and their relatives).

• Your senior is responsible for discharging patients from day surgery. Legally you are not supposed to sign discharge forms for patients until you have full medical registration.

Oro-facio-maxillary surgery

Being an House Officer for the oro-facio-maxillary surgeons usually involves rapid clerking of patients who are going to have their teeth pulled, usually their wisdom teeth. These patients are often teenagers and rarely present problems:

• Make sure you get under-16 parental consent while the parents are on ward. Otherwise you will have to bring them in from home to sign the consent form.

• Try writing and photocopying a prototype clerking sheet for these patients.

• Always ask about heart lesions and blood clotting disorders. Listen for murmurs. Have a list of antibiotics for prophylactic cover in your filofax or folder to fill into the drug chart.

• Know how to read dental shorthand for teeth:

[3] Dr Jean Miller. *Day Surgery Workshop.* Sponsored by Anglia and Oxford Regional Health Authority, 15 June 1994.

(European version)
Adults

R   8+7+6+5+4+3+2+1+|+1+2+3+4+5+6+7+8   L
   8–7–6–5–4–3–2–1–|–1–2–3–4–5–6–7–8

Children

R   5+4+3+2+1+|+1+2+3+4+5   L
      5–4–3–2–1–|–1–2–3–4–5

- Examples of teeth notation:
  The upper and lower right wisdom teeth is 8 +/8–
  The upper left wisdom tooth is +8
  The lower left wisdom tooth is –8
- Take to the bedside:
  Blood cards and bottles for FBC, U&E, INR.
  Clerking sheet.
  Drug chart.
  Consent form.
  Stethoscope.

Surgical protocol clerking sheet

Figure 15.1 is a condensed example of a surgical protocol clerking sheet that you might want to reproduce to ensure comprehensive, legible clerking. You may need to modify it to suit your particular specialty. It is also a good idea to leave plenty of space for additional comments for patients whose details are not covered by the protocol.

It is easy to photocopy the protocol directly onto your hospital's clerking forms, but you first need to make a template to photocopy from. Place a clerking form beneath some plain A4 paper and scroll both into a typewriter so that the plain paper is on top. Type out the first page of the protocol onto the plain paper so that it lines up with underlying form. Repeat for the second (and maybe third) page of the protocol. Alternatively you can use a word processor and adjust the page margins to fit the hospital forms. Load a photocopier's tray with hospital forms and photocopy the protocol onto them.

Name: .... DOB: .... Occupation: ....

Admitted for: ....

HPC: .... ☐ Weight loss ☐ Past PU
.... ☐ Change in bowel habit ☐ Alcohol intake
.... ☐ Blood in stool ☐ Smoking
.... ☐ Abdominal pain

Last meal:................................ Last menstrual period: ....

PMH .... ☐ H/T ☐ RF
.... ☐ Asthma/COAD ☐ Epil.
.... ☐ Sickle ☐ DM
.... ☐ HIV/HEP ☐ IHD
.... ☐ CVA ☐ TB

Drugs:.. Allergies: ....
....

F/SHx: .... ☐ Lives with ☐ Family diseases
.... ☐ Home help ☐ Mobility

F/E ....

R/CVs ☐ Chest pain ☐ Cough w/y/g/sputum ☐ Palps
☐ SOB ☐ PND ☐ Pillows
☐ Dysuria ☐ Frequency ☐ Incontinence
GU ☐ Urgency ☐ Stream ☐ Haematuria
☐ Froth in urine
CNS ☐ Fits/faints/funny turns ☐ Change in vision/speech ☐ Weakness
D/MSK ☐ Joint pain ☐ Rash
Other ....

| Examination | P = ... | Reg/irreg .... | BP = .../...... |
| | T = ... | RR = ... | |

General	R/CVS	Abdomen	Legs
☐ Jaundice	☐ JVP	☐ Bowel sounds	☐ SOA
☐ Pallor	☐ Apex	☐ Tender	☐ Ulcers
☐ Cyanosis	☐ Bruit	☐ Mass	☐ Skin changes
☐ Lymphadenopathy	☐ Expansion	☐ Bruit	
☐ Pitting oedema	☐ Breath sounds	☐ Shifting dullness	
☐ Clubbing	☐ PN	CNS	
☐ Rash	☐ SOA	☐ Reflexes ☐ Plantars ☐ Strength	
☐ Arcus	☐ HS	☐ Co-ordination ☐ Sensation	

Impression ....

Differential diagnosis ....

Plan ....

Fig. 15.1 Surgical protocol clerking sheet.

Chapter 16: Self care

How doctors are supposed to take care of patients without resentment if they don't take care of themselves is beyond us. Most are not taught much about self care in medical school. Look after yourself and become a more humane doctor in the process.

Accommodation

Although in practice no-one checks to see that you are living on-site, hospitals have a duty to provide you with acceptable accommodation without charge. There are national regulations governing the minimum acceptable standard which the hospital is obliged to comply with. These include:

• Your room should contain a 3 by 6 foot bed, telephone, cupboards, drawers, desk, chair, armchair, washbasin, be carpeted and have curtains. It should be regularly cleaned and heated.

• There should be a nearby bathroom and toilet, cooking facilities, a common room and on-site laundry facilities. Common areas should be regularly cleaned.

• On-call rooms should have clean sheets, a phone and a clean room. Call the Domestic Supervisor if there is a problem.

If you have a specific problem with your quarters, contact the designated 'Accommodation officer' or equivalent through switchboard. This person will also supply you with replacement light bulbs, toilet paper, etc. If the quarters *en bloc* are below standard, involve your doctors' mess and the junior doctors' committee.

Alternative careers

What if you have come all this way and you find that you don't want to be a doctor? Or you like it, but not enough to dedicate your life to it? Little known to many medics, having a medical degree opens many great doors. Chekhov, Maugham, Florey and Keats were all once doctors – to name a few.

• Medical training gives you all sorts of skills that you probably never even noticed. These include interviewing, analytic, mechanical, adversarial, communicating and observational skills, the ability to work within a hierarchy and still get what you want, sheer endurance and persistence (much prized in the workforce), experience of the human condition at its most vulnerable – and many others. Never think that these are wasted in a 'non-medical' career. Having medical training will enable you to bring something special to whatever you do.

• Having said that, *in general* we would advise doing at least your house job before saying good-bye to medicine. Many people find that they enjoy working much more than being a student. Without the house job year, it is hard to assess what it is all about. In any case, having full registration is useful if you ever wish to work in the future.

Bleep

• Pick up your bleep from switchboard. They will replace the batteries.
• If your bleep is too loud, cover the speaker with masking tape.
• If your bleep switches off too easily, tape can also be used to prevent the switch from moving.
• Leave your bleep on the ward (or switch it off) if you are not on-call, as switchboard may call you even when you are off-duty.

British Medical Association (BMA)

Becoming a member of the BMA not only brings you the *BMJ* with all the job adverts for next year, but provides advice and support in all areas of your work, leave, contracts, tax and financial planning. It is also of national importance as a negotiating body on behalf of all doctors. While the New Deal for Junior Doctors is not perfect, it nonetheless has been a major step forward in improving junior doctors' hours and re-defining appropriate duties for House Officers. Specific benefits of membership include:
1 Personal advice on contracts and terms of service.
2 Assistance and representation in disagreements with hospital management. This is becoming more important as Trusts and management try to change contracts and reduce pay. For example,

the BMA has threatened court action against trust management which has tried to cut pay, now protected under the New Deal terms. The BMA can assist with claims for overtime and additional hours.
3 Independent financial advice by salaried representatives on pensions, income protection, etc.
4 Insurance services. The personal contents policy is particularly useful (see p. 197).
5 The fee is tax deductible!

Car and insurance

You may buy your first car during your house job year. While you may need to purchase in July just prior to moving to your new job, cars are most expensive around July–August. Also, your hospital is obliged to reimburse you for moving expenses, so you do not necessarily need your own car to move.

Car insurance varies a lot. The BMA offers insurance for doctors, but it may be more expensive than you need if you have bought an old car. Probably the best thing to do is to ring local brokers who deal with many different insurance firms and who can get you the best deal for the cover you need. Many firms give a discount for young female drivers. Be aware that you can purchase third party insurance +/− fire and theft, if your car is not valuable.

Clothes (laundry/stains)

• Find out how to exchange white coats. A clean coat helps your morale and professional demeanour, although it is *not* more hygienic.

• Remove blood from washable items by soaking them in warm (not hot), soapy water with added salt, and then washing them regularly. Sponging the item as soon as possible helps too. For old stains, soak or wash the item in a soapy solution containing a few drops of ammonia or hydrogen peroxide.

• Remove blood from non-washable items by sponging with cold water. Cover silk with a paste of starch and water; allow to dry and brush off.

• Alternatively, *Stain Devils* remove most stains. You can buy them in large supermarkets or at dry-cleaning outlets. Make sure you buy the right one for the stain you have. *Stain Devils* are particularly useful for ink and ball-point stains.

• Finally, most stains can be removed with dry-cleaning. Hospitals should reimburse you for dry cleaning costs if you got the stain at work. Contact Personnel through the switchboard to find out how to apply for reimbursement.

Contacting medical colleagues

After graduation, all doctors are entered into the UK Medical Directory. This is a reasonably reliable way of tracking down friends from medical school and beyond. The Directory is available in hospital libraries and also from the General Medical Council nearest you.

Contract and conditions of service

Doctors' working conditions are laid down in the General Whitley Council Conditions of Service. More recently, the Junior Doctors' New Deal agreement has altered the rates at which overtime is paid, and stipulated the maximum hours for which you can be contracted to work. All hospitals, including Trusts, have to abide by these nationally agreed guidelines.

What you need to know about your contract

Your contract is a binding agreement, regulating your hours and conditions of service, pay, holiday and notice. It cannot be altered unilaterally by either you or your employer. In particular, under the Junior Doctors' New Deal, your pay cannot be cut, even if the hours of work are reduced.

1 Rota

Most House Officers still work a basic on-call rota (e.g. 1 in 5), meaning that they work a 40-hour working week and are also on duty every fifth night and every fifth weekend. Partial and full shifts refer to the workload during your period of work and not to the time-tabling. They do stipulate the maximum number of hours you work and the amount of time you must have off. Prospective cover means that when colleagues are away on holiday, the remaining House Officers cover the nights the missing colleague would have done. This works out equitably if everyone takes the same amount of holiday. Virtually all contracts stipulate that you cover your colleagues if they are sick. This provision does *not* give authorities power to force you to cover foreseen and notified absences such as annual leave.

2 Pay

NHS doctors' rates of pay are agreed nationally by the Doctors and Dentists' Review Body, which negotiates the annual pay increase each April. Your pay consists of a basic salary for the 40-hour week plus an additional number of additional duty hours (ADHs), depending on which rota you work. ADHs are paid at 52.1% of the basic pay rate if you work an on-call rota (Class 3); 70% if you work partial shift (Class 2) and 100% for full shift (Class 1). These rates are meant to reflect the different intensity of the work involved, although so-called 'on-call' rotas can be punishing.

• The number of ADHs are specified in your contract. They should include additions for prospective cover and for expected early starts and late finishes, such as 8 am ward rounds.

Overtime for early starts and late finishes can (in theory) be paid retrospectively. It requires your consultant to sign the appropriate claim form, confirming your extra work. In practice it can be difficult to achieve. Consultants and management may not look kindly on such claims, although this varies considerably from hospital to hospital.

• While the odd hour here or there probably does not warrant special overtime claims, if you are systematically working extra hours (for example by starting at 8 am instead of 9 and finishing at 7 instead of 5), then do not feel ashamed of asking for pay for honest work that you have done.

• *Always* document exactly (to the minute) when you start and finish work on a special 'overtime' sheet in your folder or filofax. Documentation substantially reinforces pay claims.

3 Holiday

House Officers are entitled to 5 weeks holiday/year, or two and a half weeks/6 month job.

• Try to avoid carrying leave forward. In theory, up to 4 days leave can be carried forward from the first job to the second, but this is often hard to achieve. Contact Personnel both at your current hospital and your future place of work to try to ensure you are granted the extra leave.

• Leave can be supplemented by 'in-lieu' days. Over the year you are likely to work several bank holidays and statutory hospital holidays. You can take a day off 'in-lieu' of each holiday worked or if you work over-night up to 9 am on the holiday morning.

• Find out the procedure for booking leave early. It may involve simply informing your consultant and her/his secretary, or there may be specific forms to be filled in and signed by your consultant.

4 Notice

House Officers only need to give 2 weeks notice of their intention to leave their post. However, to be eligible for full GMC registration you need to have completed 10 months as an House Officer, including 4 months of medicine and 4 months of surgery. It is not unheard of for House Officers to be given notice if the employing hospital is cutting back staff. In this unfortunate circumstance you will simply have to look for another job. However, there are often good job vacancies at short notice. Talk to the dean's office of your medical school and look in the *BMJ Classifieds* that come every week with the non-student version of the *BMJ*.

5 Leave

Compassionate leave

In the event of family or personal bereavement, paid leave will usually be given. Tell your consultant. If there is any difficulty, talk to your clinical tutor and Personnel.

Maternity (and paternity) leave

Regulations and rates of parental leave are complex, depending on how long you have worked and whether you intend to return to work. Female House Officers are unlikely to have worked for more than 1 year and, therefore, are allowed only 18 weeks unpaid leave. By comparison, doctors who have worked for longer than 1 year are entitled to 8 weeks full pay, 10 weeks half pay and up to 34 weeks of additional leave, to a total absence of 52 weeks. Doctors who have not declared intention to return to work receive fewer benefits.

• If you or your partner is pregnant or considering it, discuss the options for leave fully with your personnel department or the BMA.

• Sadly, unlike the rest of the European Union, the UK does not yet have paternity leave as an entitlement for employees. However, if you are an expectant father and need time off, it is worth discussing with your employer and the BMA.

Study leave

Pre-registration doctors are not allocated study leave other than time during the working day to attend clinical and pathology meetings. Post-registration doctors are entitled to 30 days of study leave per year.

Sick leave

Physical illness. It is still the case in most hospitals that if you are sick, your colleagues must cover you in addition to doing their own jobs. Because of this very few doctors will tell you to go home. Therefore, you *must* take control of the situation and go home if you need to. You may not be on death's door, but if you are struggling to keep up with your tasks *just go home*. The ward will cope. They might even celebrate. You are doing nobody any favours by lurking around shedding your virus and bad temper.

Mental illness. If you are struggling with mental burn out (depression, serious anxiety, grief, whatever) it is more important that you do some self diagnosis and get help and rest. Mental fatigue and illness is so common amongst doctors yet so little spoken about. It is also a cause of long-term absence and loss of self esteem which could be avoided with a bit of self care.

If you have trouble with illness of any kind, consider doing the following:

• Tell someone who loves you that you're sick/in trouble. They can help you summon up the courage to take time off and get help.

• See the hospital staff's doctor or nurse or your GP. They can help you medically and psychologically. They will give you any documentation you need (e.g. sick notes) and may be able to speak with your seniors if necessary. You are obliged to tell your consultant that you're sick (after 3 days absence). Unlike more junior colleagues, your consultant won't suffer directly if you take time off and will probably be sympathetic.

• Tell your immediate senior and the nurses on your wards so they can make arrangements for cover as soon as possible.

• Learn to care for yourself now and it will serve you throughout your life. This is preferable to a heart attack or Chronic Martyrdom Syndrome when you're 45.

Prolonged illness

Even if you fall ill on the first day of work and cannot work again, you are still entitled to sick pay equal to your full salary for 1 month. After this you will receive the usual state benefits. After completing 4 months full time work, an House Officer is entitled to 1 month of full pay and 2 months of half pay. If you fall ill towards the end of the contract and the illness continues after the time when you would have finished, you are entitled to continued sick pay as long as the illness lasts or until you have had all the sick pay you are entitled to.

6 Occupational health requirements

• Hospitals recommend that you register with a local GP, although in practice your notes will barely have caught up with you when you have to move on.

• On arrival at the hospital, the Occupa-

tional Health Department will ask about your immunization record. They may take nose or other swabs, particularly if you have worked in a different region or where there has been an MRSA (methicillin resistant *Staphylococcus aureus*) outbreak.

• Ask Occupational Health to check your HepB immunity which may have dramatically declined since immunization as a student. It should be approximately '100%'. If you do become infected with HepB you cannot be a surgeon or a specialist who does invasive work. See below for needlestick injuries.

• Contact the Occupational Health Department if you are ill for longer than 3 days. They will clear you for sick leave and may well give you some TLC in the meantime.

Doctors' mess

The doctors' mess may be a scruffy room strewn with old newspapers and coffee cups or a comfortable lounge with a coffee machine and satellite TV. Most messes run with a Mess President, Secretary and Treasurer and a variable number of committee members. If there is not much going on, organize an event and take command!

Making money for the mess

• Have regular drug lunches and charge the reps £100 to talk while you provide the catering at £50 per session.

• Organize with your colleagues and the financial people handling cremation fees for a part of each cremation fee to be given to the mess (e.g. £3).

• Hold a party. Have free drinks before 8.30 pm to make sure everyone arrives

early, or no-one will come until the pubs close.
• Ask doctors to make a regular deduction from their salary and arrange this with Personnel.

Drug representatives

Drug company representatives will approach you from time to time to try to influence your prescribing policy. You need to decide for yourself how you deal with them and their practice of bribing doctors with items and services (ranging from pens to dinners at local restaurants). Just a few tips:
• You are not obliged to spend time with drug reps. You can tell them politely that you do not have time to see them, or that you are not interested in discussing their products.
• On the other hand, you can influence drug availability by talking with company representatives. For instance, you can point out that such-and-such antibiotic would be more practical if it could be made up in solution and left in the fridge (like metronidazole) for a few hours, rather than needing to be given stat.
• Be wary of drug company literature. While some is reliable, much of it is misleading. To learn about drugs you'd be better off reading a pharmacology textbook, the *BNF* or the *Drug and Therapeutics Bulletin* which you receive free as an House Officer.

Insurance (room contents)

Probably the best room contents insurance against theft and damage is BMA-arranged insurance, because it is

designed specifically for junior doctors. Other policies may not have plans appropriate for your unusual living situation and generally cost much more.

Jobs

• Your SHO post is where the big divide begins: surgery/medicine/general practice. If you're not sure (most people aren't), 6 months of A&E is useful. Otherwise choose a general rotation. Ask your consultants, friends and older colleagues where the good jobs are.
• Network. Tell your consultant what you're hoping to do next. If you are set on a particular job or hospital, ask the consultant if he or she knows anyone there. A quick consultant-to-consultant chat is a time honoured way of securing the next post.
• Choose your referees carefully. One is usually the consultant you are currently working for. Well known professors and consultants add a little weight to your list – provided you actually know them well enough for them to write about you, and you are sure that they will say nice things!
• Application form. Make sure you get the basics right. If it asks to be typed or printed in green ink, do it. Include photographs or whatever else is requested. Don't jeopardize your chances at this early stage. Consider using recorded or registered delivery.

Curriculum vitae

It's probably easiest to type out your CV yourself so you can make small changes as necessary. Use high quality paper. Your consultant's secretary might oblige.

• Make sure you spell-check your CV – or proof read it carefully for misspellings. Read your CV aloud to make sure that it does not contain any disastrous sentences or factual errors.

• Try to be concrete about what you want to do. People love hearing concrete plans that are easy for them to imagine. If you know what your planned career is, say so. Put 'Career objective: chest medicine' at the top of your CV under your name.

• Make the most of your experience, listing skills you have acquired and responsibilities you have taken. Don't forget skills such as computing and languages. Make sure you include honours or prizes, even from school.

• Avoid one-word interests such as 'Reading'. Try to be concrete in demonstrating what you have done. For example, instead of saying 'Running', you might specify your running activities: 'Participation in Anglia regional running events, club secretary'.

• Create your CV so it shows you as you want to be seen. CVs are not shopping lists, nor are they confessions. If you did badly one year you can minimize the fact in how you present your CV. Just make sure that you don't say things that are blatantly untrue, and that you include certain professional details (see later).

• When asking for a reference, supply your referee with a current CV and brief outline of achievements you want them to mention.

• Show your CV to your Mum or a close friend to make sure that you haven't left anything important out. Consider showing it to your present colleagues/consultant and secretaries who have probably seen many CVs and can give you good advice on both content and style.

• If the form you are given for your CV is inadequate, staple your CV to it, unless the instructions strictly state otherwise.

A CV should include (at least):

Personal: name, address, nationality, date of birth, civil status, interests, brief general education, and non-medical employment (if any).

Medical: undergraduate education including medical school, date of entry and graduation, honours or prizes, qualifications, previous and present appointments, career plans, publications, society memberships, referee names and telephone and fax numbers.

The interview

• Try to visit the hospital before the interview, see the department and meet the consultants. If you have already met some of the interview panel you may be more relaxed.

• Follow the basics: clean suit, hair and shoes, be punctual and courteous.

• Find out from the person co-ordinating the interview what you can expect inside the interview room, such as how many interviewers you will face and the expected length of the interview.

• Early questions are likely to focus on your CV and experience. Be prepared to discuss and expand on anything you have mentioned. At this level it is rare that you will be asked medical questions. Be prepared for questions about your career plans. Try to say something concrete, even if you are unsure about your future career. At all costs avoid looking aimless. Ethical issues such as euthanasia may be discussed.

• Listen attentively to the interviewers' questions and take care to answer them directly rather than blurring the issue. Don't ramble.

• While remaining relatively formal, don't be afraid to be yourself. If the interviewer doesn't like you as you really are, you probably don't want to work for them anyway.

• Write thank you letters to your referees for their help and support. You may need them again in the future!

Consultant career prospects

The medical and dental staffing prospects are published annually in the journal *Health Trends*, published by the Department of Health. The prospects include the current number of SRs, consultants, likely consultant vacancies and future consultant numbers, by specialty. The journal should be in your medical library; if not, ring the Department of Health in London.

Locums

Locums pay well if you can bear working through your holidays and weekends.

• Get registered with one or more locum agencies. These are advertised in the *BMJ Classifieds*. Medical personnel at your hospital will know the name of local agencies. Note that different agencies pay very different rates. Shop around.

• Try to negotiate travel expenses with the agency.

• If you secure a locum at a hospital you don't know, the following is a checklist of things to do when you arrive:

1 Sign in at the switchboard. Sign-in registers what time you arrive at the hospital – the locum agency may check when working out your pay.

2 From switchboard and reception, pick up: bleep, keys, map of the hospital, identification (if necessary) and essential telephone numbers:
   • A&E.
   • Admissions.
   • Biochemistry (and on-call bleep number).
   • Haematology (and on-call bleep number).
   • Porters.
   • Wards.
   • Radiology department (and on-call bleep number).

3 Find out (on the hospital map) where these are:
   • Blood gas machines.
   • Canteen.
   • Doctors' residence.
   • Drink machine.
   • ITU.
   • Radiology department.
   • Wards.

4 Bleep your senior and arrange to meet.

5 Dump your overnight bag in the doctors' residence.

6 Go to the wards and introduce yourself.

7 On the wards, stuff a folder (see p. 7) with: blood forms, history sheets, consents, fluid charts, drug charts, X-ray forms. Clip the phone numbers to the front of the folder.

8 Locate IV equipment, catheters, drug cupboard, resuscitation equipment.

9 Find out:
- Who gives IV drugs.
- If there is a phlebotomist in the morning and where to leave requests.

10 If possible, speak to the person who usually carries your bleep about any useful information s/he may know about patients, staff and the hospital.

11 If you are required to attend a ward round when you should have finished the locum, you are entitled to extra hours' pay; contact the locum agency as soon as possible about this. If you have to leave on the dot, let your senior know this from the outset.

12 Hospitals that are desperate to fill locums will often negotiate terms with you, such as allowing you to arrive late or leave early if necessary.

Meals

- Try not to miss meals. Twenty minutes for a hot evening meal makes little difference to patient care, but it will keep *you* going.
- Don't forget to drink as much liquid as possible. It's easy to get dehydrated and even more tired when you're too busy to stop for tea-breaks.
- If canteen food is awful, take in microwave meals. It's comforting to have a treat such as fruit or a chocolate bar.
- Find out about local take-aways. Some may discount hospital staff. There are almost always people on the shift who will share a meal with you and cut down the delivery cost.

Medical defence

Historically, it was compulsory to belong to a defence organization for representation and insurance against medicolegal complaints arising out of the care of patients. This changed in 1990 when Crown Indemnity came into force, so that the Crown, or rather the NHS employer, will pay the costs of investigation and damages for cases arising during your employment with them. However, protection under Crown Indemnity is limited. It does *not* cover incidents arising outside the hospital, such as 'good Samaritan' acts, nor private practice. Most importantly, Crown Indemnity may not support you if you have a conflict with your employer. The advantages of joining a medical defence organization are expert, round-the-clock advice with *your* interests at heart. The overall benefits of the various organizations (e.g. MDU, MPS) are similar, so join whichever one appeals.

Money

For the first time, your bank account will be filling up with a £1000 or so each month. Be a bit careful. It's not unusual for people to run up thousands of pounds of credit card debts – and to spend the next few years paying them off.

Income protection if long-term sick or disabled

Various organizations offer income protection (also known as PHI or Permanent Health Insurance). On payment of a monthly premium, you are covered for prolonged absence, even if you never work again. If you have a mortgage and family, sickness cover becomes more important. Research the various policy options carefully.

Payslip deductions

National Insurance is a compulsory contribution which will pay for your future state pension, maternity pay and sick leave.

Superannuation is not compulsory but is essential for your pension. The national state pension is meagre. The NHS superannuation scheme is your employer's scheme to allow you to make additional pension contributions. You contribute 6% and the NHS contributes a further 4% of your basic salary (before tax and ADH additions).

• You have to sign a form at the start of your job stating your intention to stay with or opt out of the superannuation scheme. The only people who might not want to contribute towards their own superannuation are those who are pretty sure that they will not be working for long in the NHS, such as foreign graduates. However, NHS superannuation can be accrued to other public sector positions in the UK such as the civil service and university posts.

• Your can reclaim superannuation contributions if you have worked for the NHS for *less than 2 years*. Otherwise your contributions will stay locked in the scheme.

• Think long and hard before leaving the superannuation scheme to join a private pension plan. It is highly unlikely that you could ever match the security and returns of the NHS scheme.

Pensions

As described above, the superannuation scheme provides the main pension for doctors. When you retire, your benefits are an annual pension of up to half your salary and a lump sum of three times your annual pension. The exact calculations are:

Pension = years of service/40 × pensionable salary

Pensionable salary = highest annual salary earned in any of the 3 years prior to retirement

• Few doctors complete the full 40 years of service that would allow them to receive the maximum possible pension. However, it is possible to make additional contributions to your future pension. The most cost-effective way is to make Additional Voluntary Contributions (AVCs) into the NHS Group Scheme, administered by the Equitable Life. This is a well-kept secret, with low commission and charges. You should contact your local Equitable Life Representative or write to the Equitable Life Assurance Society, Group Voluntary Contributions Department, PO Box 183, Walton Street, Aylesbury, Bucks HP21 7QW. It is also possible to buy 'added years', as if you had worked for longer than you really have.

• You will doubtless meet financial salesmen who will offer to sell you Free Standing AVCs, i.e. a way of investing your contributions in their company's policies (and earning them a bonus). Be aware that your whole first year's contribution may disappear in the salesperson's commission.

• Your expenses as a young doctor may

be high – with a new house, a car and possibly a family. As long as you are aware that you should consider further pension contributions at some date, these need not be a priority in your first year of work (whatever financial advisers may say).

Tax

Earning a regular salary unfortunately means paying serious tax. You will save time, trouble and money if you make an effort to keep basic records. Each month you should get a payslip giving details of your pay, national insurance, and any other deductions you have authorized such as telephone bills or car parking charges. Check this to see you have not been overcharged.

A P60 is sent to you at the end of the tax year (5 April). It is your record of how much income you have received and tax you have paid. A P45 is given to you when you leave the job, to take to the finance department at your next job to show how much tax you have been paying. If you lose it you will probably be taxed the wrong amount (usually overtaxed) until the tax office sorts it out – which may take months.

Understanding your tax

Doctors have tax deducted automatically from their pay before they receive it (known as PAYE – Pay As You Earn). The Inland Revenue works out how much tax you are likely to owe throughout the year and this is deducted monthly from your salary.

House Officers start work in August, part-way through the tax year which runs from 6 April to 5 April. This means that your first pay cheque will be larger than any of the subsequent months. The tax year ends on 5 April. After this your tax office will send you a note stating how much tax you paid in the last year, and how much tax you ought to pay in the next year (P60). You could just leave it there. However, it is quite likely that you have been overtaxed and could claim money back on tax deductible items. You also have a duty to declare untaxed income so that it can be taxed. At the simplest, you could just write a letter declaring your tax deductible items and untaxed income; alternatively contact your tax office for a full tax return form. Your personnel department will be able to give you full details of your tax office, which is usually determined by where you work.

Tax deductible items (on which you can reclaim money you have paid in tax) include:

1 GMC fee (but only the renewal fee, not the initial joining-up fee).
2 Medical defence subscription.
3 BMA membership.
4 Replacement of medical equipment (e.g. better stethoscope).
5 Medical journals.
6 New books to replace old editions.

In later years, membership to one of the Royal Colleges is also tax deductible.

Untaxed income which must be declared

The main item here is cremation fees ('ash cash'), worth approximately £40, which you receive for completing part 1 of the cremation form. In recent years the Inland Revenue has tightened up on this potential evasion. It is not unknown for them to investigate funeral directors' records and compare them with doctors' tax returns. Non-declaration constitutes tax evasion and is penalized accordingly. You should declare full cremation fees even if there is a deduction, for example for mess expenses. Other untaxed cash payments such as the fees for completing other forms should also be declared.

Tax allowances

Everyone has a personal allowance, i.e. an amount of income they can earn before being taxed. In **1997/8** you earn £4045 before paying tax. The next £4100 is taxed at 20%; the next £22 000 is taxed at 23%. The highest rate of 40% is paid on any income above this (i.e. when you earn more than £30 145 per annum). This will not apply to House Officers unless you have substantial additional income.

If you are married you can also claim the married person's allowance which allows a further slice of income to be taxed at 20%. In 1997/8 this allowance was £1830. For historical reasons it is allocated initially to the husband, but it can now be allocated to either partner, or split equally between them. Fill out the relevant form from your tax office.

Telephone banking

Consider switching to telephone banking, which can be accessed 24 hours a day from your phone. Telephone banks allow you to withdraw cash from a regular bank's ATM machines, but do all other transactions by phone and registered post. Many banks now offer telephone services. *Which* magazine regularly reviews banking services so look out for the next *Which* report. At the time of going to press (February 1998), the most highly regarded bank in our circle of medical friends was the Co-op Bank which is open from 6am to 12pm for telephone banking but has the benefit of linking your credit card to your current account so that you can move money around very easily. In addition, they give £10 to Amnesty International (you never know when you may need them!) when you take out an account and pay 0.1% of all your credit card transactions to charity. PC or what?

Needlestick injuries

If you needlestick yourself, do the following:

1 Squeeze blood from the site immediately. Go to a sink. Continue to squeeze blood from the wound under fast running, warm water.
2 Don't panic. Virtually all doctors needlestick themselves from time to time and very, very few have contracted anything undesirable, even from patients infected with HIV and hepatitis.
3 If they consent to it and are counselled about the implications of having an HIV test done, take one clotted (brown) tube of blood from the patient. This needs to be analysed immediately for HIV and hepatitis.
4 Alert your senior and/or the public health unit in the hospital. They will instruct you further. They will require you to do the following, depending on patient status.

If the patient is known to be HIV-positive

• Don't panic. Thousands of HIV needlestick injuries have resulted in only a handful of cases of HIV worldwide. The chances of your getting HIV are very small. On the other hand, don't give yourself a hard time if you do panic. Almost everyone does, and people who haven't stuck themselves with HIV infected blood just don't understand what this is like. Seek help from a counsellor or GP if you are suffering from excessive anxiety about it.

1 Have one clotted tube of blood taken from yourself. Give it to the public health unit/GP for storage. This is to ascertain your hepatitis/HIV status at the time of injury. It will only be analysed in the unlikely event that you are later found to be positive.

2 After 3 months (at least) have an HIV check. Over 95% of people who are going to seroconvert do so within 3 months. If this is negative, repeat it at 6 months and 1–2 years. The second test will give you peace of mind.

3 Use condoms at least until the 3 month check.

4 Having HIV tests does not usually pose a problem for getting life insurance (as it once did) if you explain that you are a health professional having a routine HIV check. However, if you are concerned, you can usually have your blood checked confidentially by your virology lab or the hospital's STD clinic (so it will not be recorded in your medical records). The latter is preferable, as you will get proper counselling for the test.

If the patient is known to be hepatitis-positive

1 Follow your doctor's instructions. Give the lab a clotted sample of your blood as soon as possible after injury to ascertain your hepatitis antibody status at the time of injury.

2 Find out what kind of hepatitis the patient has. They may have chronic hepatitis from lupus which is not infective. If they have Hep B, you may need instant immunoglobulin; if they have Hep C you may need interferon treatment.

3 You may need to be re-tested for hepatitis antigen after 6 months. In the meantime, it is advisable to practise safe sex.

Not coping

You are not alone. *Everyone* has disastrous days, weeks months and even years. Everyone thinks about giving up medicine. If you feel like chucking it all in, this does not mean that you are less motivated or committed than anyone else. In fact the chances are that if you are feeling like that, so is everyone else, except that they'd rather die than admit it. Group studies suggest that when one person is feeling lonely, isolated, alienated and generally miserable, it is much more likely that others in the environment are too. Studies show that a substantial proportion of junior doctors become clinically depressed; most suffer depression and anxiety at least a few times during their career.

• Confidential counselling services have been established which provide counselling for doctors who are not coping. The

BMA can advise you where such services are and how to contact them.

• Make sure that you do not blame yourself for structural problems in your workplace that have nothing to do with you. For instance, a bullying consultant or charge nurse will make anyone's life hell, not just yours. Consider talking to others – or even to your local BMA rep – about such problems, before taking it all upon yourself.

• Everyone experiences considerable turbulence upon entering the workplace. Remember that feeling low or anxious may just be manifestations of adjusting to a completely new way of life, and will pass within a few months, however painful they seem at present.

• Simple fatigue can greatly exacerbate mental distress. If you are feeling miserable, try going to bed really early on your nights off.

Part-time work (flexible training)

• It is now possible to be a part-time House Officer. At present part-time House Officer jobs are individually negotiated and created by postgraduate tutors. Part-time usually means half time, doing half the number of on-call nights. Unfortunately, the corollary of doing half time is that you must be an House Officer for 2 years instead of one.

• It is possible to continue flexible part-time training as an SHO, up to and including consultant level. At Registrar level and above, national recognition and approval for part-time training is required. At SHO level, simple agreement with the Postgraduate Dean suffices.

• In rare cases, part of the House Officer year can be spent in general practice.

Representation of junior doctors

You can get a great deal done if you and your colleagues work together on agreed goals. You can act as a body in several ways:

Doctors mess, mess president and committee. This may meet regularly or on an ad-hoc basis. It usually has several roles: organization of social events, representation of junior doctors' interests to management, administration of mess funds, rooms, etc.

Junior doctors' division. This is usually a hospital committee which meets every few months to discuss issues relevant to junior doctors. The main frustration for House Officer representatives is that you rarely work at the hospital long enough to see changes implemented.

New Deal committee. Hospitals should have convened this committee or something similar to consider and implement the issues arising from the Junior Doctors' New Deal, i.e. reducing doctors' hours and delegating inappropriate duties.

BMA. Junior doctors may stand as BMA representatives for local, regional and national committees. You should be allowed a reasonable amount of time off to attend to these activities. In practice it is usually doctors beyond the House Officer year who have the career stability to embark upon medical politics.

Sleep

Those who have not been sleep deprived cannot understand what it's like to be obsessed by the thought of sleep. Admittedly the situation has much improved since the 1980s. However, you can get very run down if you don't take care of yourself.

• If you've had little or no sleep the night before, a shower and breakfast go a long way to prevent the awful grey feeling of fatigue.

• Ask someone else to hold your bleep for a few hours. Have a nap at lunch time in an on-call room.

• After long shifts, go to bed, go directly to bed, do not pass Go, do not collect £200! You will be grateful the next morning.

• Another trick is to sleep in a side room while on call. This radically cuts down time getting up and travelling across car parks and long corridors to the ward, and rarely results in more calls. In the morning you only have to get up minutes before the ward round. Always strip your own sheets in the morning.

Appendix A: Useful tests, numbers and other information

Addresses

The British Diabetic Association, 10 Queen Ann Street, London W1M 0BD (Tel: 0171-323 1531)

British Medical Association (and *BMJ*), BMA House, Tavistock Square London WC1H 9JP (Tel: 0171-387 4499)

Central Public Health Lab, 61 Colindale Avenue, London NW9 5HT (Tel: 0181-200 6868)

Communicable Disease Surveillance Centre (for notifying diseases), 61 Colindale Avenue, London NW9 5DF (Tel: 0181-200 6868)

Disabled Living Foundation (for advice on equipment), 380–384 Harrow Road, London W9 2HU (Tel: 0171-289 6111)

General Medical Council, 178 Portland Street, London W1N 6JE (Tel: 0171-580 7642)

Health Information Line (for doctors & patients) (Tel: 0800-665544)

Medical Defence Union, 3 Devonshire Place, London W1N 2EA (Tel: 0171-486 6181)

Medical and Dental Defence Union, Macintosh House, 120 Blythwood Street, Glasgow G2 4EH (Tel: 0141-221 5858)

Medical Protection Society, 50 Hallam Street, London W1N 6DE (Tel: 0171-637 0541)

Medical Sickness Society (Tel: 0181-866 1924)

Multiple Sclerosis Society, 25 Effie Road, London SW6 1EE (Tel: 0171-610 7171)

Poisons Information

Belfast	01232-240 503
Birmingham	0121-507 5588
	0121-507 5589
Cardiff	01222-709 901
Dublin	00353-1-837 9964
	00353-1-837 9966
Edinburgh	0131-536 2300
Leeds	0113-243 0715
London	0171-635 9191
	0171-955 5095
Newcastle	0191-232 5131

Barthel score

The Barthel score helps you to assess quickly whether someone can manage at home. It is particularly useful at social rounds. A total score of 15 or more is 'good'.

Bathing
0   dependent
1   independent (bath and shower, in and out)

Bladder
0   incontinent or catheterized and unable to cope alone
1   occasional incontinence (1/day)
2   fully continent

Bowels
0   incontinent
1   occasional incontinence (1/week)
2   fully continent

Dressing
- 0   dependent
- 1   needs some help (e.g. with buttons, laces)
- 2   independent

Feeding
- 0   dependent
- 1   needs some help (e.g. with cutting)
- 2   independent (food within reach)

Grooming
- 0   dependent (hair, teeth, shaving)
- 1   independent

Mobility
- 0   immobile without help
- 1   independent with wheelchair (includes turning)
- 2   walks with one person assisting
- 3   independent

Stairs
- 0   dependent
- 1   needs assistance (physical, verbal, mechanical)
- 2   independent (up and down)

Toilet
- 0   dependent
- 1   needs some help
- 2   independent (transfer, wiping, dressing)

Transfer
- 0   unable (cannot balance to sit)
- 1   needs major assistance (2 people) but can sit
- 2   needs minor assistance (physical or verbal)
- 3   independent

Glasgow Coma Scale

Eyes open
- 4   spontaneously
- 3   to voice
- 2   to pain
- 1   none

Verbal response
- 5   oriented
- 4   confused
- 3   inappropriate words
- 2   incomprehensible words
- 1   none

Motor response
- 6   obeys command
- 5   localizes to pain
- 4   withdraws
- 3   flexes
- 2   extends
- 1   none

Total (out of 15)
Serious: ≤8
Moderate: 9–12
Mild: 13–15

Mental Health Act

1 Always get senior advice before using the Mental Health Act.

2 Section 4 states that for an emergency admission, the nearest relative *or* an approved Senior Nurse *or* a social worker *or* a doctor *as well as* the medical recommendation of one doctor who must have seen the patient within the previous 24 hours, can apply for 72 hours of compulsory admission on the grounds of:
- Urgent necessity.
- Mental disorder requiring hospital admission.
- Danger to him/herself or others.

3 Section 5(2) states that a patient already in hospital as a voluntary patient can be detained for 72 hours under the same conditions as Section 4, except that it only requires a single medical recommendation by the doctor in charge of the patient's care, *or* another doctor on the staff of the hospital who is nominated by the doctor in charge.

4 Sectioning a patient does not permit you to treat a concurrent physical condition unless it is life threatening.

Mini-mental test score

There are several versions of the mini-mental test score. This is one of them. It gives you a quick, ball park measure of someone's mental state. This can be very useful in casualty or in the middle of the night. Falstein's full mental test score is outlined in the *Oxford Handbook of Clinical Medicine* (see p. 2).

1 What month is it?

2 What year is it?

3 Where are you now?

4 Recall an address (have the person repeat this after you and then ask it from them at the end of the other questions).

5 Name three objects (e.g. pen, hand, watch).

6 What is your name?

7 Start of World War I (1914) or World War II (1939)?

8 Name of the current UK monarch.

9 Name of the Prime Minister.

10 Count backwards from 20 to 1 without an error.

• When giving the patient an address to recall, use one that you know so that *you* remember it. There is nothing more embarrassing than failing your own mini-mental test score!

• Questions 7–9 are culturally specific. They can be substituted for questions the patient is likely to know.

Notifiable diseases

Doctors are legally required to report notifiable diseases to their local medical officer for environmental health. The microbiology department know who this is, as do people at the town hall. Alternatively you can contact the Communicable Disease Surveillance Centre: 61 Colindale Avenue, London NW9 5EQ (Tel: 0181-200 6868, 0181-965 1118).

Recognized notifiable diseases are those listed below.

Anthrax

Cholera

Continued fever (Scotland only)

Dysentery

Ebola virus disease

Encephalitis (England, Northern Ireland only)

Erisypelas (Scotland only)

Food poisoning (England, Scotland only)

Gastroenteritis in infants <2 years (Northern Ireland only)

Infective hepatitis (Northern Ireland only)

Infective jaundice (England only)

Leprosy (England, Scotland only)

Leptospirosis

Malaria (England, Scotland only)

Measles

Membranous croup (Scotland only)

Meningitis (acute)

Meningococcal septicaemia

Mumps

Ophthalmia neonatorum (England, Scotland only)

Paratyphoid fever

Plague

Poliomyelitis

Puerperal fever (Scotland only)

Rabies
Relapsing fever
Scarlet fever
Smallpox
Tetanus (England only)
TB (England, Northern Ireland only)
Typhoid fever
Typhus
Viral haemorrhagic fever
Viral hepatitis
Whooping cough
Yellow fever

Results

The following are normal ranges for results of tests. However every lab is different; make sure that you use their values, particularly for unusual tests which require local calibration of lab equipment.

Consider copying the results that are important for your job onto a single sheet which you can stick at the back of a folder or filofax for easy reference.

Haematology

APTT (factors VIII, IX, XI, XII)	35–45 seconds
Eosinophils	0.04–0.44 (1–6%) × 10^9/l
ESR female	(age + 10)/2
ESR male	(age)/2
FDPs	lab dependent
Hb (male)	13.5–18 g/dl
Hb (female)	11.5–16 g/dl
Lymphocytes	1.3–3.5 (20–45%) × 10^9/l
MCV	76–96 fl
Monocytes	0.2–0.8 (2–10%) × 10^9/l

Neutrophils	2–7.5 (40–75%) × 10^9/l
Platelets	150–400 × 10^9/l
Prothrombin (INR) (factors I, II, VII, X)	10–14 seconds (expressed as ratio versus control. Normal INR is 1.0)
RCC (female)	3.9–5.6 × 10^{12}/l
RCC (male)	4.5–6.5 × 10^{12}/l
Reticulocytes	0.8–2% (25–100 × 10^9/l)
WCC	4–11 × 10^9/l

Biochemistry

Acid phosphatase (prostate)*	0–1 IU/l
Acid phosphatase (total)*	1–5 IU/l
ACTH	3.3–15.4 pmol/l
ADH	0.9–4.6 pmol/l
Albumin	35–50 g/l
Aldosterone	100–500 pmol/l
Alk phos	30–300 IU/l
Alpha fetoprotein*	<10 IU/l
ALT	5–35 IU/l
Amylase	0–180 U
Angiotensin II	5–35 units
AST	5–35 IU/l
Bicarbonate	24–30 mmol/l
Bilirubin	3–17 μmol/l
Ca (ionized)	1–1.25 mmol/l
Ca (total)	2.12–2.65 mmol/l
Chloride	95–105 mmol/l
Cholesterol	3.9–7.8 (>5 is high) mmol/l
Cortisol (am)	280–700 nmol/l
Cortisol (pm)	140–280 nmol/l
Creatine kinase (males)	25–195 IU/l
Creatine kinase (females)	25–170 IU/l
Creatinine	70–150 μmol/l

CSF glucose	>2/3 of plasma glucose
Ferritin	20–300 μmol/l
Folate	5–6.3 nmol/l
FSH	2–8 U/l
GGT (males)	11–51 IU
GGT (females)	7–33 IU
Glucose (fasting)	4–6 mmol/l
Glycosylated Hb*	6–8.5%
Haptoglobin	20–125 μmol/l
Iron (male)	14–31 μmol/l
Iron (female)	11–30 μmol/l
LDH	240–545 IU/l
Mg	0.75–0.15 mmol/l
Osmolality	278–305 mOsm/kg
PTH	<0.1–0.7 μg/l
Phosphate	0.8–1.45 mmol/l
Potassium	3.5–5.0 mmol/l
Prolactin (males)	<450 units
Prolactin (females)	<600 units
Protein (total)	60–80 g/l
Red cell folate*	0.36–1.44 μmol/l
Sodium	135–145 mmol/l
TSH	0.5–5.7 U/l
T_4	70–140 nmol/l
Thyroxine (free)	9–22 pmol/l
TIBC*	54–75 μmol/l
Triglyceride	0.55–1.9 mmol/l
T_3	1.2–3.0 nmol/l
Urea	2.5–6.7 mmol/l
Uric acid (males)	210–480 μmol/l
Uric acid (females)	150–390 μmol/l
Vitamin B_{12}	0.13–0.68 nmol/l or >150 ng/l

Arterial blood gases

pH	7.35–7.45
Pao_2	>10.6 kPa
$Paco_2$	4.7–6.0 kPa
Base excess	+/−2 mmol/l
Bicarbonate	22–26 mmol/l
Type 1 respiratory failure	$Pao_2 < 8$; $Paco_2 < 6$
Type 2 respiratory failure	$Pao_2 < 8$; $Paco_2 > 6$

Useful biochemical formulae

$$\text{Anion gap} = (Na + K) - (Cl + HCO_3)$$
$$= 4\text{–}17 \text{ mmol/l}$$

• The anion gap is made up of ions such as phosphate, sulphate, lactate.
• It is high in any condition with reduced clearance or excess production of any unmeasured anions (e.g. DKA, lactic acidosis).
• It is low in hyperalbuminaemia, liver disease and paraproteinaemias.

Corrected calcium = reported total Ca
$+ 0.2 \times (40 - \text{the actual albumin})$

Creatinine clearance (males)
$$\frac{1.23 \times (140 - \text{age}) \times \text{wt (kg)}}{\text{creatinine}}$$

Creatinine clearance (females)
$$\frac{1.04 \times (140 - \text{age}) \times \text{wt (kg)}}{\text{creatinine}}$$

* Clotted tube.

Fitness to drive

Condition	Normal licence	Notification of DVLC	Vocational licence
Anaesthetic	Avoid for 48 hours post-general anaesthetic	No	
Angina, chronic and stable	Avoid driving if symptomatic while driving	No	Many restrictions; refer to DVLC
Angioplasty	1 month	No	Check with DVLC
Aortic aneurysm	No restrictions	Yes	Permanent ban
Arrhythmias	If symptomatic while driving. Driving may continue once symptoms are controlled	Yes	Check with DVLC
Occasional ventricular premature beats	No restrictions	No	
Frequent or polymorphic premature beats	Stop driving, pending CVS investigation	Yes	
Ventricular tachycardia	Stop driving, pending CVS investigation Driving may continue once symptoms are controlled *with* annual review	Yes	
Implanted defibrillator	Avoid driving forever	Yes	
CNS disorders	Where definite diagnosis of progressive disability; refer to DVLC for specific advice with consent of patient	Yes	Check with DVLC

	Driving forbidden until 1 month after pacing	Yes	Forbidden
Complete heart block			
Conduction abnormalities	If symptomatic avoid driving pending CVS investigation. Can drive when symptoms are controlled	Yes	Check with DVLC
Congenital heart anomalies	No restrictions unless arrhythmia, angina or syncope. Post-surgery, 1 month	No No	Check with DVLC
Congenital heart block (usually bradycardia)	3 year licence after CVS investigation, including stress test and 24-hour ECG, repeated annually	Yes	Usually forbidden
Diabetes	Can hold licence for 1, 2 or 3 years depending on complications and diabetic type. IDDM patients need to demonstrate: • Understanding of disease • Reasonable control • No frequent or unexplained hypoglycaemic attacks Always carry sugar in car	Yes	Need to notify DVLC if becomes IDDM, with individual review Established IDDM will not be granted new vocational licences
Drugs (if any side effects which impair consciousness or motor response)	Avoid driving while taking drug Warn patient that alcohol potentiates side effects of many drugs	No	
Epilepsy	Can hold (renewable) licence for up to 3 years if: • Free of fits for 2 years • Fits only while asleep for 3 years • Avoid for 6 months during treatment changes	Yes Yes Yes	Allowed if fit free since 5 years of age or Fit free for 10 years and off medication and seeing neurologist annually to confirm fit-free status

Fitness to drive (*Cont.*)

Condition	Normal licence	Notification of DVLC	Vocational licence
Single fit	• Cannot drive until investigated • Possible 1-year ban	Yes	See previous comment for driving post-fit
Hypertension (uncomplicated)	No restriction	No	
Impaired locomotor system	Avoid driving. If permanent disability, refer to DVLC	Yes	Refer to DVLC
MI	Avoid driving for 1 month	No	Many restrictions; refer to DVLC
Pacemakers	Can ho'd licence for up to 3 years 1 month post-implantation *if*: • Followed up annually • Asymptomatic	Yes	Refer to DVLC
PVD	No restriction		
Syncope, TIA, LOC	Avoid driving until problem solved; 3 month ban	Yes	Permanent ban
Valvular heart disease	No restrictions if no arrhythmia, angina or syncope	No	Check with DVLC

From Raffel A. (ed.) (1985) *Medical Aspects of Fitness to Drive: a Guide for Medical Practitioners.* Medical Commission on Accident Prevention, London.

Appendix B: Diagrams for explaining procedures to patients

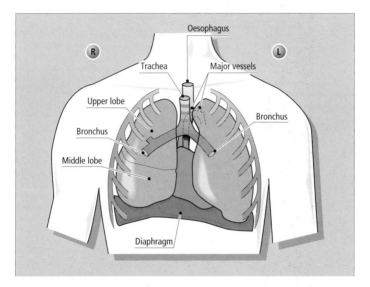

Fig. A1 The thorax. For example:
• Bronchoscopy.
• Chest surgery.

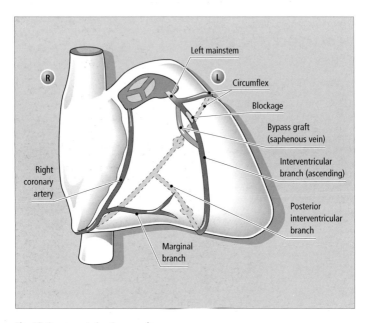

Fig. A2 Coronary arteries. For example:
• CABG.

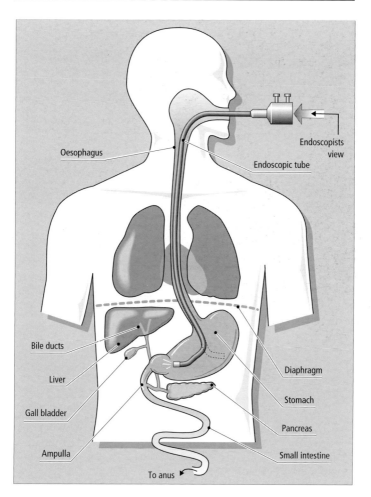

Fig. A3 Upper gastrointestinal tract. For example:
- Upper endoscopy (± ERCP).
- Liver biopsy.
- Cholecystectomy/biliary surgery.
- Pancreatitis.
- Gall stones.

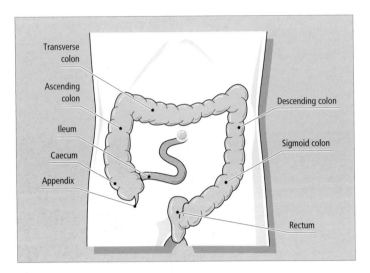

Fig. A4 Large intestine. For example:
- Colonoscopy.
- Large bowel surgery.
- Diverticular disease.
- Colonic carcinoma.

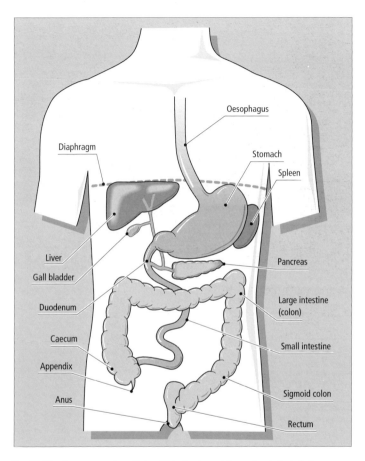

Fig. A5 Digestive organs – schematic (small intestine is much longer than indicated). For example:
- Major abdominal surgery.
- Intestinal disorders.

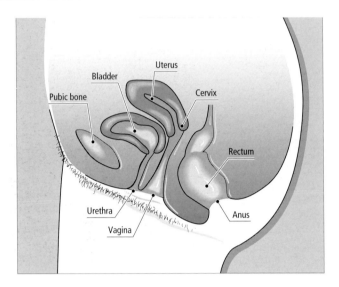

Fig. A6 Female pelvis. For example:
• Catheterization.
• Gynaecological disorders.

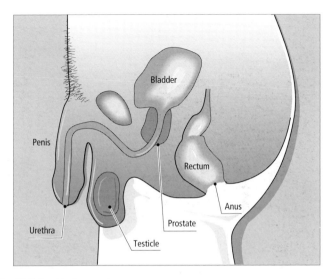

Fig. A7 Male pelvis. For example:
- Catheterization.
- Prostatectomy.

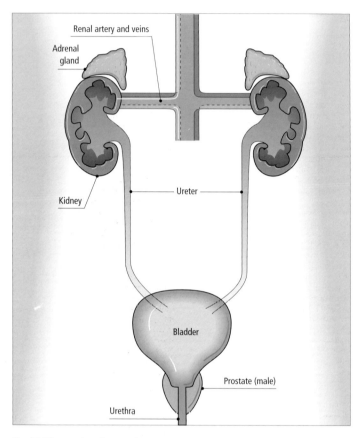

Fig. A8 Urinary system. For example:
- Renal biopsy.
- Renal stones.
- Bladder disorders.

Index

abdominal pain 36–7
pain relief 131
   pregnant women 109
abdominal plain film 173–4
abdominal surgery 183
accident and emergency 15–20
   admitting patients 15–16
   medical conditions 16
   pain relief 20
   patient information organization
     16
   surgical conditions 20
accident forms 10–11, 53, 54
accommodation 191
ACE inhibitors 74
acetylcysteine (Parvolex) 18
acid–base disorders 71, 136–7
acidosis 72, 137
acupuncture 130
acyclovir 111
Addison's disease 75, 80
addresses 207
adenosine 41
ADH-secreting tumour 81
admitting A&E patients 15–16
adrenal insufficiency 66
adrenaline 68
albumin deficit 41
alcohol withdrawal 45, 54, 57, 104–5
alcoholism 104–5
alkalosis 75, 76, 137
allopurinol 54
alternative careers 191–2
amiloride 74
aminoglycosides 56, 83
aminophylline poisoning 19
amiodarone 39, 102
amitriptyline 69
amoxycillin 100
amphetamines overdose 57
amphotericin B 75
ampicillin 99
amputation 183
anaemia 37–8
   blood transfusions 81

   differential diagnosis 37
   investigations 38, 123
anaesthetic risk 182
anaesthetics 183–4
anal fissure 46
anaphylaxis 67, 71, 78, 82, 102–3
   management 68
angina 43
anion gap 137, 211
antacids 37, 42, 46, 47
antibiotics 55, 56, 74, 99–100, 188
   peri-operative prescribing 181
   post-splenectomy 183
   side effects 47, 48, 54, 55, 100
anticholinergics poisoning 19
anticoagulation 63, 64
   peri-operative prescribing 181
   protocol 100–1
antidiarrhoeal agents 48
anti-emetics 72
antihistamines 70
antipyretics 55
anuria 83–4
anxiety 66, 68, 69
aortic aneurysm 36, 43, 44
   repair 183
aortic dissection 43
apologies 27
appendicitis 36
arrhythmia 38–41
   bradycardias 39–40
   hypokalaemia 75
   hypotension 67
   initial management 38–9
   moribund patient 70
   normal heart rate 39
   tachycardias 40–1
arterial blood gases 133–8
   arterial puncture procedure 135–6
   arterial puncture sites 134
   normal values 136
   pH 136–7
   Po_2 136
   type 1 respiratory failure (pink puffers)
     138

arterial blood gases (*cont.*)
    type 2 respiratory failure (blue bloaters)
       138
arteriography 176
ascites
    intravenous fluids 58, 61
    investigations 122
    sites for tapping 163
aspiration pneumonia 100
aspirin 126, 131
    poisoning 17, 19
asthma 79
atrial fibrillation 39, 40, 49
atrial flutter 40, 49
atrial tachycardia 49
atrioventricular (AV) heart block 39
atrioventricular (AV) nodal rhythm 49
atropine 40, 133, 165

bad news 85–6, 87
    information for patients' families 30–1
bank nurse 29
barium enema 175
barium meal 175
barium swallow 175
Barthel score 207–8
basal cell carcinoma 78
basic emergency routine 84
bed allocation 16
benzodiazepines 65, 69
bereavement officer 91
beta-blockers 39
bibliographic databases 22–3, 24
biliary surgery 183
biochemistry, results 210
bisacodyl 47
bladder catheterization 64, 138–40
    men 138–9
    women 139–40
bladder washout 83, 84
bleep 192
blood cross-match, surgical patients 179, 180
blood cultures 140
blood forms 11
blood requests 11
blood samples
    arterial blood gases 133–4
    children 105
    from central lines 147
    haemophiliacs 107
    HIV/AIDS patients 107–8
    venous sampling procedure 140–2

blood stains 3, 193
blood transfusion 54, 55, 75, 81–2
    anaemia 37
    upper gastrointestinal bleeds 60, 61
blue bloaters 138
bone pain relief 131
books 2
bowel infarction 54
bowel resection 182
brachial artery puncture 134
bradycardia 39–40
British Medical Association (BMA) 192
    junior doctor representatives 205–6
    newspaper cuttings database 25
British National Formulary (BNF) 94
bulk-forming agents 47
bullous skin lesions 77
bupivacaine 155, 158

CAGE questionnaire 104
calcitonin 42
calcium 41–3
    corrected 41, 211
calcium channel blockers 39, 46
calcium gluconate infusion 43, 75
calcium resonium (polystyrene sulphonate
    resin) 75
candidiasis 100, 108, 110, 111
cannulae sizes 143
cannulation 142–4
    clearance of blockages 144
    indications 144
    right internal jugular vein 146
    subclavian vein 146
car 192
carbamazepine 18, 102, 131
carbenicillin 75
cardiac arrests 32–4
    protocol 33–4
cardiology investigations 120–1
cardioversion 40, 41
carotid sinus massage 41
CD-ROM 21
cefuroxime 100, 102
cellulitis 100
central lines 144–9
    approaches 144, 146
    blocked lumen 147
    CVP measurement 148, 149
    indications 144
    insertion 144–7
    sepsis 147

temporary/tunneled lines 147–9
central pontine myelinosis 81
central retinal vein/artery occlusion 52
central venous pressure (CVP) measurement
    148, 149
cephalosporin 99, 100
cerebrovascular accident (CVA) 45, 57, 67
    head CT 176
cervical carcinoma 62
charge nurse 29
chest drains 149–51
    indications 150
    insertion 150–1
    removal 151
chest infection 100
chest pain 43–4
chest X-ray 173
    pre-operative 184
children 105
    consent 105, 182, 188
    dental charting 190
    oro-facio-maxillary surgery 188, 190
chloral hydrate 69
chlormethiazole 45, 57, 104, 105
chlorpheniramine 68, 70, 81, 82
chlorpromazine 45
chlorpropamide 80
cholecystitis 36, 43
Christian Scientists 109
chronic obstructive airways disease (COAD)
    73, 78, 79
Chvostek's sign 43
cimetidine 47
ciprofloxacin 100
cirrhosis 59, 69
clinical stalemate 113
Clostridium difficile 47, 48, 99, 122
clotrimazole 111
cluster headache 64
Cochrane Database of Systematic Reviews
    (CDSR) 23, 25
co-codamol 132
codeine 48, 64, 66, 128, 131
    side effects 130
co-dydramol 131
colchicine 47
colloid fluid replacement 60, 61, 71
colonic surgery 183
colonoscopy 117
colostomy 182
common calls 35–84
communication 26–31

bad news 30–1, 85–6, 87
    consultants 27
    GPs 27–8
    nurses 28–9
    patients 29–30
    patients' families 30–1
    senior registrars 27
    terminal care 85–8
    see also information-giving
communications software 23, 24
computerized tomography 176
computers 21–4
    hardware 21–2
    Internet 23–4
    on-line database access 23
    software 22–3
concussion 45
conditions of service 193–6
confidentiality 31
conflicts management 27
confusion 44–6, 68, 69
conjunctivitis 52
consent 181–3
    children 105, 182, 188
constipation 46–7
consultants
    career prospects 199
    communication 27
contract 193–6
    compassionate leave 195
    cover 193
    holiday entitlement 194
    maternity/paternity leave 195
    notice 194–5
    occupational health requirements 196
    overtime 194
    pay 194
    prolonged illness 196
    rota 193
    sick leave 195–6
    study leave 195
contrast studies 173–5
controlled drugs 95–6
controlled percentage face masks 73
coping problems 204–5
co-proxamol 64, 132, 188
corneal ulceration 52
coronary arteries 216
coronary artery spasm (variant angina) 51
coroner 91–2
costochondritis 43
counselling services 204

cover for absence 193, 195
crash calls 32–4
creatinine clearance 211
cremation 92
cremation fees 92, 196
   tax 202–3
cremation forms 90, 92–3
critical appraisal 25, 26
curriculum vitae 197–8
Cushing's disease/syndrome 121
Cushing's reflex 67
cyclizine lactate 72
cyclobenzaprine 66
cytotoxic agents 47, 72, 80

daily patient notes 10
danthron decusate 47
databases 23, 25
day surgery 188
   clerking 188, 189
death 89–93
   clinical confirmation 89
   cremation forms 92–3
   informing relatives 90
   referral to coronor/procurator fiscal 91–2
   registration 90
   statistics 93
   what to do 89–90
death certificate 90–1
   occupation-related deaths 91
   war-related deaths 91
deep vein thrombosis (DVT) 54, 55
defibrillator 32
dehydration 42, 46, 47, 48, 66, 68
dementia 45
dental charting 188, 189
depression 66, 68, 69, 108
   in doctors 195, 204
   patient care 106
desk-top publishing 23
diabetes mellitus 54, 55, 56, 61, 62
   drug dilutants 96
   investigations 121
   neuropathy 131
   surgery 185–7
      GKI (glucose potassium insulin) regime 186
      insulin infusion 186–7
      protocols 186
diabetic ketoacidosis (DKA) 36, 58, 62, 74
diamorphine 78, 129, 130, 131
diarrhoea 47–8, 75

   investigations 48, 122
diazepam 45, 46, 57
diclofenac 20, 131
diflusinal 126
digestive organs 219
digoxin 39, 40, 75
   administration protocol 101
   side effects 47, 65, 72, 101
   therapeutic drug levels 102
digoxin toxicity 41
   electrocardiogram 51
dihydrocodeine 128, 131
diphenhydramine 73
disabilities assessment 4–5
discharge 6
   day surgery 188
   GP communication 27–8
   information for patients' families 30
discharge plan 4, 5, 113
discharge summary 12–13, 27–8
disseminated intravascular coagulation (DIC) 123
distress 26
diuretics 75, 106
diverticulitis 36
doctors' mess 196–7, 205
docusate sodium 47
domperidone 72
dopamine agonists 72
dopamine infusions 96
doxapram 73
dress 3
Dressler's syndrome 43
droperidol 72
drug abbreviations 35
drug administration 96–9
   infusions 96–7
   intravenous drugs 98–9
drug charts 94–5
   continuous infusions 97
   verbal requests 96
drug effects
   anaphylaxis 102–3
   confusion 45
   constipation 46
   diarrhoea 47
   falls 53
   fever 54
   headache 64
   hyperkalaemia 74
   hypokalaemia 75
   hyponatraemia 80

hypotension 67
itching 70
nausea/vomiting 72
oliguria/anuria 83
rashes 76
drug prescribing 94–6
    abbreviations 95
    children 105
    controlled drugs 95–6
    infusions 97
    pre-emptive 103
    pre/peri-operative 181
    pregnant women 109
    TTO/TTA 12
    verbal requests 96
    written prescriptions 95
drug representatives 197
drug vials opening 96
drug withdrawal 57
drugs 94–103
dry skin 70
dysmenorrhea 63–4

ectopic pregnancy 63
eczematous skin lesions 77
elderly patients 106
    confusion 44
    falls 53, 54
    intravenous fluids 58
    overflow diarrhoea 47
    sedation 69
electrocardiogram (ECG) 48–52
    atrial fibrillation 48, 49
    atrial flutter 49
    atrial tachycardia 49
    AV nodal rhythm 49
    basic parameters 48–9
    calculating axis 49, 50
    common diagnoses 48
    lead placement 151, 152
    myocardial infarction 51
    P waves 49
    PR interval 49–50
    pre-operative 184
    procedure 151–2
    pulmonary embolism 51–2
    QRS complexes 51
    ST segment 51
    T waves 51
    ventricular tachycardia 49
electrolyte imbalance
    acid-base disorders 137

confusion 45
crash calls 32
elderly patients 106
fits 57
intravenous fluids 58
nausea/vomiting 72
electrolytes, body fluids 59
emergency routine 84
Emla anaesthetic cream 143
empyema 80
    chest drains insertion 150, 151
encephalitis 65
endocarditis, subacute bacterial (SBE) 55–6,
    140
    investigations 120–1
endocrinological investigations 121–2
endometriosis 63
Entonox 129
epilepsy 56
equipment 3–4, 15
erythematous skin lesions 77
erythromycin 99, 100
evidence-based medicine 25–6
examination of medical patient 113, 115
exercise stress test 152–3
exsanguinating bleed 32
eye complaints 52–3
    acute red eyes 52
    floaters 53
    sudden loss of vision 52

face masks
    facial bruising 74
    oxygen therapy 73
falls 53–4, 69
families
    communication 30–1, 87
    consent for post mortem 90
    informing of patient's death 90
fatigue
    doctor 26, 35, 36, 195, 204–5
    post-operative 182
female pelvis 220
femoral artery puncture 134, 135
fentanyl 181
ferrous sulphate 46
fever 54–6, 57, 58, 82
fibroids 63
firm timetable 8
fitness to drive 212–14
fits 56–7
flexible training 205

floaters 53
flucloxacillin 56, 74, 100
fluconazole 111
fluid overload 58, 80
    central venous pressure (CVP) 149
forced expiratory volume (FEV) 166
forced vital capacity (FVC) 167
forms 7
    accident and emergency 15
    information management 11–12
    serial 12
fractures 53, 54, 106
frusemide 78, 81

gastritis 36, 37, 43, 72
gastroenterological investigations 122
gastrointestinal bleeds
    investigations 122
    lower GI tract 61
    upper GI tract 59–61
genito-urinary surgery 183
gentamicin 100, 102
geography of hospital 4
GKI (glucose potassium insulin) regime 185, 186
Glasgow Coma Scale 208
glaucoma, acute 52, 65
glucose abnormalities 61–2
glucose administration 75
glucose tolerance test 153
glyceryl trinitrate (GTN)
    continuous infusions 96
    sublingual 43, 44
GP liaison 27–8
    accident and emergency admissions 15, 27
    death 89–90
    discharge summary 12, 13, 27–8
    potassium supplements 76, 106
    self-discharge 14, 27
granisetron 72
grief 19, 26, 106
Groschong IV catheters 147
gynaecological disorders 62–3

Haemaccel 61, 71
haematology
    investigations 122–3
    results 210
haematuria 64
haematemesis 59, 60, 61
haemoglobinopathies 37
haemophiliacs 107

haemorrhoids 46
haemorrhoidectomy 183
haemothorax 150–1
haloperidol 45, 46, 80
handbacks 13
handovers 13
handwriting 26
    drug charts 94
head injury
    head CT 176
    skull X-ray 174
headache 64–6
    pain relief 65, 131
    post-lumbar puncture 160
heart block 39, 50, 51
heart failure 40, 66, 78, 79
    central venous pressure (CVP) 149
    congestive 80, 83
heparin 100, 101
    arterial blood samples 134
hepatitis B 133
    haemophiliacs 107
    immunization status 196
    needlestick injuries 204
hepatitis C
    haemophiliacs 107
    needlestick injuries 204
hepatitis testing 203, 204
herpetic keratitis 52
Hickman catheters 147
history taking
    medical background 112, 114
    medical patients 112–15
    surgical patients 178
    systematic (functional) enquiry 113, 114
HIV testing 108
    confidentiality 108, 204
    following needlestick injuries 203, 204
HIV/AIDS
    fever 56
    haemophiliacs 107
    medical problems 108
    needlestick injuries 203–4
    patient care 107–8
    taking blood 107–8
Hodgkin's lymphoma 70
holiday entitlement 194
5-HT$_3$ antagonists 73
hydrocortisone 42, 68, 81, 82, 111, 187
hyoscine butylbromide 131
hypercalcaemia 41–2, 46
hyperglycaemia 52, 57, 61, 62

hyperkalaemia 74–5
hyperparathyroidism 41
hypertension 66
    investigations 120
    malignant 66
hypertensive encephalopathy 65
hyperthyroidism 40, 54
    investigations 122
hyperventilation 79
    spurious hypocalcaemia 42
hypoalbuminaemia 41
hypocalcaemia 42–3
hypoglycaemia 45, 57, 61–2, 71
hypokalaemia 46, 75–6
    elderly patients 106
    potassium replacement 76
hypomagnesaemia 76
hyponatraemia 58, 80–1
    correction 80–1
hypoparathyroidism 42
hypotension 67–8
hypothermia 39, 106
hypothyroidism 39, 46, 80
    investigations 121–2
hypovolaemia
    central venous pressure (CVP) 149
    hypotension 67
    oliguria/anuria 83
    upper gastrointestinal bleeds 59, 60
hypoxia 44, 45, 57, 79
    arterial blood gases 136
    elderly patients 106

ibuprofen 54, 64, 66, 74, 126, 131
ileostomy 182
ileus 46
immunization status 196
immunocompromised host 56
    diarrhoea 47, 48
    fever 54, 55, 56
income protection 200
infection
    antibiotic treatment 100
    confusion 45
    diarrhoea 47, 48
    fever 54, 55
    hypotension 67
    moribund patient 71
    nausea/vomiting 73
    oliguria/anuria 83
    with steroid therapy 110
    tachycardia 40

inflammatory bowel disease (IBD) 47, 54
inflammatory skin lesions 77
information-giving 29
    breaking bad news 85–6, 87
    confidentiality 31
    consent for surgery 181–2
    day surgery 188
    diagrams 215–22
    HIV testing 108
    patients' families 30–1
    preparation for procedures 116, 133
        see also specific procedures
    radiology 171
initiative 2
injections 154
    intramuscular 154
    joint 157
    subcutaneous 154
insomnia 68–9
insulin therapy
    diabetic surgical patients 185, 186–7
    hyperkalaemia 75
    hypoglycaemia 61, 62
    hypokalaemia 75
insurance 192, 197, 200, 204
intensive therapy unit (ITU) 181
intercostal block 155
internal jugular vein cannulation 146
Internet 21, 23–4
interpreters 37, 86
interstitial renal disease 80
intestinal fistula 75
intestinal infarction 36
intestinal obstruction 36, 37, 46, 72
intracranial pressure elevation 39, 65, 67, 72
intramuscular injections 154
intrauterine contraceptive device (IUCD) 63
intravenous drugs administration 98–9
    liquid drugs 98
    powdered drugs 98, 99
intravenous fluids 58–9
    children 105
    elderly patients 106
    hyponatraemia 80
    inadequate potassium replacement 75
    Na/glucose composition 59
    prescription 58
    terminal care 88
intravenous urography 173–4
investigations
    anaemia 38, 123
    cardiology 120–1

investigations (*cont.*)
  diarrhoea 48, 121
  endocrinology 121–2
  gastroenterology 122
  haematology 122
  medical patient 120
  neurology 123–4
  normal result ranges 210–11
  renal medicine 124
  respiratory medicine 124–5
  rheumatology 125
Ipecac 19
iritis, acute 52
irritable bowel syndrome (IBS) 46, 47
ischaemic heart disease (IHD) 43, 44
  investigations 120
isoprenaline 40
itching 69–70

jaundice 39, 70
  surgical patients 185
Jehovah's witnesses 109
job interviews 198–9
jobs 197–200
  consultant career prospects 199
  interviews 198–9
  referees 197, 198, 199
joint aspiration 155–7
joint injections 157
junctional (nodal) supra-ventricular
        tachycardia 40
Junior Doctors' New Deal 192, 193
  hospital committee 205
junior doctors' respresentation 205

ketoconazole 108

lactulose 47
lap-top computer 22
laparoscopic surgery 182
laryngospasm 42, 43
laxatives 46, 47, 48, 103
lecturer practitioner 29
legal aspects 10
  confidentiality 31
  consent 181–2
  day surgery case discharge 188
  drug charts 94, 95, 96
  falls 53
leukoerythroblastic anaemia 38
lice 70
lignocaine 155, 156, 157, 158, 163

  with adrenaline 158
literature
  evidence-based medicine 25–6
  keeping up to date 24–5
lithium 102
liver biopsy 118
liver failure
  drug dilutants 96
  intravenous fluids 58, 61
  investigations 122
local anaesthesia 157–8
locums 199–200
long-term illness income protection 200
loperamide 48
lorazepam 46
lower gastrointestinal tract 218
  bleeds 61
  investigations 122
lumbar puncture 158–60
  bloody tap 160
  headache following 160
  indications/contraindications 158

Macintosh computers 21–2
macular skin lesions 77
magnetic resonance imaging (MRI) 176–7
male pelvis 221
malignant disease
  fever 54
  hypercalcaemia 41, 42
  hyponatraemia 80
malignant hypertension 66
malnutrition in elderly 106
Mantoux test 161
marcaine 158
marking surgical patients 184
mastectomy 183
maternity leave 195
meals 200
Med 3 form 14
medical defence 200
medical patient
  examination 113, 115
  history taking 112–15
  management planning 115–16
  preparation for procedures 116–20
  specialist referrals/investigations 120–5
MEDLINE 23, 25
mefenamic acid 64
melaena 59, 60
melanoma 78
meningism investigations 123

meningitis 57, 65, 66, 72
Mental Health Act 208–9
   self-discharge prevention 14
   treatment refusal 19
mental illness in doctors 195–6
meprobamate 131
metabolic disorders
   confusion 45
   constipation 46
   fits 57
   hyperkalaemia 74
   nausea/vomiting 72
methylprednisolone 157
metoclopramide 72, 78
metronidazole 56, 100, 102
miconazole 108, 111
migraine 64, 65, 66, 72
mineralocorticoid deficiency 75
mineralocorticoid excess 75
mini-mental test 20, 45, 53, 209
mithramycin 42
modem 21, 23, 24
money management 200–3
   income protection 200
   payslip deductions 201, 202
   pensions 201–2
   tax 202–3
monitor 22
moribund patient 70–1
   differential diagnosis 71
   emergency routine 84
morphine 128, 129, 130, 131
   continuous infusions 96
motor dysfunction 53
Mycobacterium tuberculosis 161
myeloma 123
myocardial infarction 39
   abdominal pain 36
   atrial fibrillation 40
   central venous pressure (CVP) 149
   chest pain 43, 44
   crash calls 32
   electrocardiogram 51
   fever 54
   hypotension 67
   investigations 120
   moribund patient 70
   nausea/vomiting 72
   pain relief 131
   shortness of breath 78, 79

naloxone 71, 130

naproxen 128, 131
nasal specs 73
nasogastric tube insertion 161–2
National Insurance 201
nausea/vomiting 71–2
needlestick injuries 203–4
nephrotic syndrome 80
   investigations 124
nerve blockade 130
netilmycin 100
neurological investigations 123–4
   moribund patient 71
nicotine 40, 104
nifedipine 66
night calls 35–6
night rounds 5–6
night sedation 102
nitrates 40, 65
nitrous oxide/oxygen 129
nodal (junctional) supra-ventricular
      tachycardia 40
nodular skin lesions 77
non-steroidal anti-inflammatory drugs
      (NSAIDs) 72, 74, 83, 126, 128, 129
   pros/cons 129
'not for resus' 32
notes, patient 10
   breaking bad news 86
   death 89, 90
notice 194–5
notifiable diseases 209–10
nurse manager 29
nurses
   communication 28–9
   drug administration 96, 97
   grades 28–9
   shifts 28, 29
   verbal drug requests 96
nystatin 108, 111

obstructive lung disease 73, 78, 79
   investigations 124
occult bleeding
   gastrointestinal blood loss 37, 38
   hypotension 68
oesophageal spasm 43, 44
oesophageal varices 59
oesophagitis 43
oliguria 82–4
   differential diagnosis 83
ondasetron 73
on-line database access 23

ophthalmic examination 3, 52
ophthalmoscope 3
opiate overdose 19
    moribund patient 70–1
opiates 103
    antidote 130
    bolus injection 129–30
    constipation 46
    infusions 130
    nausea/vomiting 72
    oral 128
    pain relief in addicts 20
    post-operative hypotension 68
    pros/cons 130
    respiratory depression/confusion 45
    terminal pain relief 88
optic neuritis 52
oral contraceptive pill 63, 100, 181
oral hypoglycaemic agents 61, 62
    diabetic surgical patients 185, 186
organization of paperwork 7–8, 16
orientation day 1
oro-facio-maxillary surgery 188–9
overdose 16–20
    aspirin 17, 19
    fits 57
    history taking 19–20
    Ipecac 19
    opiates 19, 70–1
    paracetamol 17–19
    patient assessment 17, 19–20
    patients refusing treatment 19
    poisons information 17
    washouts 19
overtime 194
oxazepam 69
oxygen therapy 73–4
    chronic obstructive airways disease
        (COAD) 73
    face masks 72–3
    nasal specs 73

P6 computers 22
P45 202
P60 202
P waves 49
pacemakers
    check before cremation 89, 92
    insertion 118–19
pain
    acute/chronic 128
    associated symptoms 45, 46, 47, 72
        elderly patients 106
        emotional component 128
        physical component 127–8
        stimulus-independent 127–8
pain relief 126–32
    abdominal pain 37
    accident and emergency 20
    common clinical conditions 131
    dysmenorrhea 63
    headache 65
    hypertension 66
    insomnia 69
    mild pain 131
    moderate pain 131
    opiate addicts 20
    oral drugs 126, 128
    renal colic 20
    severe pain 131
    terminal care 86, 88
pancreatitis 36, 42, 43, 72
Papaveretum 129–30, 131
paperwork organization 7–8, 10–14
papular skin lesions 77
papulosquamous skin lesions 77
paracentesis (peritoneal tap) 162
paracetamol 55, 66, 82, 103, 131
    pros/cons 129
paracetamol poisoning 17–19
    Parvolex (acetylcysteine) 18
paraprotein investigation 123
paroxysmal atrial tachycardia 40
part-time work 205
Parvolex (acetylcysteine) 18
paternity leave 195
patient communication 29–30
patient information management 7, 8,
        11 12, 16
pay 194
payslip deductions 201, 202
peak expiratory flow rate (PEFR) 168, 169
pelvic inflammatory disease (PID) 63
penicillin allergy 99
penicillins 83, 99
pensions 201–2
Pentium computers 21, 22
peptic ulcer 36, 37, 43, 72
pericardial tamponade 32, 70, 78, 79, 149
pericarditis 43, 51
peritoneal tap (paracentesis) 162
peritonism 36, 72
personal folder 7
pethidine 129, 131, 165

phaeochromocytoma 121
phantom limb pain 131
pharmacists 94, 95
phenobarbitone 42, 57
phenothiazines overdose 57
phenytoin 42, 57, 102
phlebitis 74
pigmented skin lesions 77
pink puffers 138
piperacillin 56
plain films 173
platelet transfusions 82
pleural aspiration 155, 156, 162–5
    indications 163
    procedure 164
pleural effusion
    chest drains insertion 150–1
    investigations 125
pleuritic chest pain 43, 131
    intercostal block 155
pneumonia 36, 40, 43, 78, 79
    investigations 124
pneumothorax 32, 43, 44, 71, 78, 79
    chest drains insertion 150
poisons information 17, 207
Police Officers 31
polyarthritis investigations 125
polycythaemia rubra vera 70
polystyrene sulphonate resin (calcium
    resonium) 75
porphyria 80
post mortem 90
post-operative care 184–5
    haemophiliacs 107
post-operative confusion 45
post-operative fever 54
post-operative hypertension 67
post-operative hypotension 68
post-operative ileus 46
post-operative pain relief 131
    day surgery 188
potassium 74
    hyperkalaemia 74–5
    hypokalaemia 46, 75–6
        elderly patients 106
    replacement 75, 76
        oral 76
    supplements 74, 76, 106
PR interval 49–50
pregnancy 36, 62–3, 72
    patient care 109
    radiology 173

pre-operative checklist 184
pre-operative hypertension 66
presenting complaint 112
press information 31
priority setting 2
procedures 133–70
    diagrams for patient explanations 215–22
prochlorperazine 72, 165
procurator fiscal 91–2
professionalism 26
prostatectomy 183
pseudo-membranous colitis 47, 99
psoriasis 76
psychiatric disorders 19–20, 45
pulmonary embolism 32, 40, 43, 44, 54, 66,
    71, 78, 79
    central venous pressure (CVP) 149
    electrocardiogram 51–2
pulmonary oedema 71, 78
pulse oximetry 74
pulsus paradoxus 165
purpuric skin lesions 77
pustular skin lesions 77

QRS complexes 51

radial artery puncture 134
radioactive implants, check before cremation
    89, 92
radioisotope scanning 177
radiology 171–7
    arteriography 176
    computerized tomography 176
    contrast studies 174–5
    magnetic resonance imaging (MRI) 176–7
    patient preparation 171, 173
    plain films 173–4
    pregnant women 173
    radiation exposure 171, 172
    radioisotope scanning 177
    requests 171
    ultrasound 175–6
ranitidine 60, 111
rash 76–7, 82
referees 197, 198, 199
referral letters 13–14
renal biopsy 119–20
renal colic 20, 131
renal failure 66, 69
    acute 75
    investigations 124
renal investigations 124

renal parenchymal disease 64
respiratory failure
    investigations 125
    type 1 (pink puffers) 138
    type 2 (blue bloaters) 138
respiratory function tests 165–9
respiratory investigations 124–5
results, normal ranges 210–11
retinal detachment 52
retroperitoneal bleed/abscess 36
rheumatoid arthritis 54
rheumatological investigations 125
rib collapse 43
rota 193

safe sex 204
salbutamol 68, 78
salicylates poisoning 19
sarcoid 42
scabies 70
sciatica 131
sedation
    confusion 45, 46
    falls 53, 54, 69
    insomnia 69
    night 102
self-care 191–206
    terminal care 87, 89
    work environment 15
self-discharge 14
self-discharge note 14
senior registrar communication 27
senna 47
septicaemia 100
serial forms 12
sharps disposal 15, 28, 108, 133
shingles 43, 52, 66, 70, 76
shock 40, 54
shortness of breath 78–9
'sick cell' syndrome 81
sick leave 195–6
    prolonged illness 196
sick notes 14
sick patient checklist 80
sick sinus syndrome 39
sickle cell anaemia 109–10
    pre-operative testing 181
    sickle crisis 109
sigmoidoscopy 117
sinus bradycardia 39
sinus tachycardia 40
sinusitis headache 65

sister 29
skin lesions 76–7
    disease categories 77
skin tumours 77
skull X-ray 173, 174
sleep 206
slides preparation 23
Slow K 46, 76
small bowel enema 175
social security benefit 14
social-work rounds 4
sodium 80
    hyponatraemia 58, 80–1
        correction 80–1
sodium valproate 102
software 22–3
'special' nursing 29
spinal cord compression/lesions 46
spirometry 166, 169
spironolactone 74
splenectomy 183
spreadsheets 23
squamous cell carcinoma 77
ST segment 51
staff nurse 29
stains 3, 193
staphylococcal infection 56, 74, 77
steroid conversions 103
steroid therapy
    acute illness management 111
    anti-inflammatory steroid equivalent doses
        110
    face masks use 74
    joint injection 156, 157
    patient care 110–11
    peri-operative prescribing 181
    side effects 48, 110 11
    surgical cover 187
    withdrawal 111
sticky labels 178
stool softeners 47
streptococcal skin infection 77
stroke 176
student nurse 28
study leave 195
subarachnoid haemorrhage 57, 65, 160
    head CT 176
subclavian vein cannulation 146
subcutaneous injections 154
subdural haematoma 45, 57, 65
subtalar joint aspiration 157
suicidal thoughts 106

HIV/AIDS patients 108
    patient assessment 19–20
sulphonamides 83
superannuation 201
supra-ventricular tachycardia (SVT) 40–1
surgical patients 178–90
    anaesthetics 183–4
    clerking 178–81, 188, 189
    clerking sheet 189, 190
    consent 181–3
    day surgery 188
    diabetes mellitus 185–7
    expected side effects of surgery 183
    haemophiliacs 107
    history sheet 178
    jaundice 185
    marking 184
    oro-facio-maxillary surgery 188–9
    peri-operative prescribing 181
    post-operative care 184–5
    pre-operative checklist 184
    steroid dependent 187
    theatre lists 184
    thyroid surgery 187–8
sutures 169–70
    removal 169
        haemophiliacs 107
sympathomimetics 40
syncope 53, 54
syndrome of inappropriate ADH (SIADH)
        80, 81

T waves 51
tachycardia 40–1
tax 202–3
    allowances 203
    tax deductible items 202
    untaxed income declaration 92, 202–3
team nursing 28, 29
telephone banking 203
telephone numbers 7, 8, 9
temazepam 69, 103, 181
temporal arteritis 52, 65, 66
tenoxicam 128
tension headache 64, 65, 66
tension pneumothorax 72, 149
terfenadine 70
terminal care 85–9
    breaking bad news 85–6, 87
    communication 85–8
    pain control 86, 88
    prescribing 88

self-care 87, 89
    support organizations 88–9
    symptom control 88
thalassaemia 37
theatre lists 184
theophylline 40
therapeutic drug levels 102
thiazide diuretics 42, 47, 80
thioridazine 80
thorax 215
threatened miscarriage 63
thyroid function investigation 121–2
thyroid surgery 187–8
    expected side effects 183
ticarcillin 75
tobramycin 102
total parenteral nutrition (TPN) 42, 43
tracheostomy 183
transcutaneous electrical nerve stimulation
        (TENS) 130
transfusion reactions 54, 55, 81, 82
transient ischaemic attack (TIA) 45
trauma
    confusion 45
    fits 57
    hyperkalaemia 74
treatment refusal 109
    overdose 19
triamcinolone 157
triamterene 74
tricyclic antidepressants
    overdose 19, 57
    side effects 46, 64
trimethoprim 100
tropicamide 3
TTA 12
TTO 12
tuberculosis 42
    investigations 124–5

UK Medical Directory 193
ultrasound 175–6
unconscious patient
    investigations 123–4
    overdose 17, 19
untaxed income declaration 202–3
upper gastrointestinal bleeds 59–61
    high risk patients 59, 60
    low risk patients 61
upper gastrointestinal endoscopy 116–17
    complications 117
upper gastrointestinal tract 217

upper gastrointestinal tract (*cont.*)
   investigations 122
urinary retention 36, 45, 83
urinary system 222
urinary tract infection (UTI) 64, 72
   antibiotic treatment 100
   investigations 124
   recurrent 124
uterine carcinoma 62

vaginal bleeding 62–3
vancomycin 100
   therapeutic drug levels 102
variant angina (coronary artery spasm) 51
vascular skin reactions 77
ventricular extrasystoles 39, 51
ventricular tachycardia (VT) 40, 41, 49, 50
verapamil 46
vertebral collapse 43
vesiculobullous skin lesions 77
villous adenoma 75
visual loss, sudden 52
vitamin B$_{12}$ deficiency 37

vitamin D deficiency 42
vitamin D intoxication 42
vomiting 72, 75, 76

wandering atrial pacemaker 39
ward calls 35–6
ward rounds 4–5
   discharge plan 113
   history/examination summary 113
   post-operative care 184–5
ward sister 29
warfarin 100, 101
   arterial blood samples 134
   face masks use 74
washouts 19
white coat 192–3
wisdom teeth extraction 188
Wolff–Parkinson–White syndrome (WPW)
   40
   PR interval 50
word processing 22
work environment 15
wound abscess 36

NOTES